GUILFORD SUBSTANCE ABUSE SERIES

Editors

HOWARD T. BLANE, Ph.D.
Research Institute on Alcoholism, Buffalo

THOMAS R. KOSTEN, M.D.
Yale University School of Medicine, New Haven

venting AIDS in Drug Users and Their Sexual Partners
L. SORENSEN, LAURIE A. WERMUTH, DAVID R. GIBSON,
G-HEE CHOI, JOSEPH R. GUYDISH, and STEVEN L. BATKI

Alcohol in Human Violence
KAI PERNANEN

king and Driving: Advances in Research and Prevention
R. JEAN WILSON and ROBERT E. MANN, Editors

iction and the Vulnerable Self: Modified Dynamic Group Therapy for Substance Abusers
EDWARD J. KHANTZIAN, KURT S. HALLIDAY, and WILLIAM E. McAULIFFE

cohol and the Family: Research and Clinical Perspectives
R. LORRAINE COLLINS, KENNETH E. LEONARD, and JOHN S. SEARLES, Editors

Children of Alcoholics: Critical Perspectives
MICHAEL WINDLE and JOHN S. SEARLES, Editors

roup Psychotherapy with Adult Children of Alcoholics:
tment Techniques and Countertransference Considerations
MARSHA VANNICELLI

Psychological Theories of Drinking and Alcoholism
HOWARD T. BLANE and KENNETH E. LEONARD, Editors

Alcohol and Biological Membranes
WALTER A. HUNT

roblems in Women: Antecedents, Consequences, and Intervention
SHARON C. WILSNACK and LINDA J. BECKMAN, Editors

inking and Crime: Perspectives on the Relationship between Alcohol Consumption and Criminal Behavior
JAMES J. COLLINS, JR., Editor

Date Due

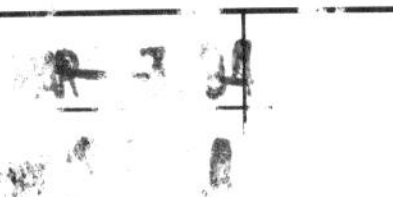

Preven

in Drug

Their Sex

THE

Pre

JAMES

KYUN

Dri

Add

Al

C

Tre

Alcohol I

Dr

Preventing AIDS

in Drug Users and Their Sexual Partners

JAMES L. SORENSEN, LAURIE A. WERMUTH,
DAVID R. GIBSON, KYUNG-HEE CHOI,
JOSEPH R. GUYDISH, AND STEVEN L. BATKI
University of California, San Francisco

THE GUILFORD PRESS
New York London

Published by The Guilford Press
A Division of Guilford Publications, Inc.
72 Spring Street, New York, NY 10012

Printed in the United States of America

This book is printed on acid-free paper.

Last digit is print number: 9 8 7 6 5 4 3 2 1

Library of Congress Cataloging-in-Publication Data

Preventing AIDS in drug users and their sexual partners /
James L. Sorensen . . . [et al.].
p. cm.—(The Guilford substance abuse series)
Includes bibliographical references and index.
ISBN 0-89862-173-9
1. AIDS (Disease)—Prevention. 2. Intravenous drug abuse—Health aspects. I. Sorensen, James L. II. Series.
[DNLM.1 Acquired Immunodeficiency Syndrome—prevention & control. 2. Sex Behavior. 3. Sex Counseling. 4. Substance Abuse. Intravenous. WD 308 P943]
RA644.A25P753 1991
614.5'933—dc20
DNLM/DLC
for Library of Congress 91-24707
CIP

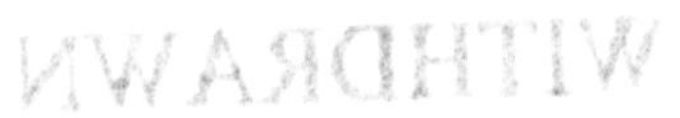

It is rather for us, the living, to be dedicated here to the unfinished work they who fought here have thus far so nobly advanced . . . for us to be here dedicated to the great task remaining before us.

—Abraham Lincoln
Gettysburg Address, November 19, 1863

Many dedicated staff members in drug treatment programs are working to minimize the problems of AIDS for their patients and to help them recover from the problems of drug abuse. Since we began working in this area, many of our coworkers have "burned out" and left the field, become ill, or died. Not all the departures and deaths are due to HIV infection, but certainly almost all are linked to the stresses and strains of working with the problems of drug abuse. We dedicate this book to our colleagues who have died since we began this effort.

Arnold Abbott
Bill Granfors
Richard Heaphy
Sam Keller
Seretta Marshall
Mark Ryan
Tom Smith

Contributors

STEVEN L. BATKI, MD, is an Associate Clinical Professor and Medical Director of Substance Abuse Services at San Francisco General Hospital, Department of Psychiatry, University of California, San Francisco.

JOSEPH A. CATANIA, PhD, is an Assistant Research Psychologist at the Center for AIDS Prevention Studies, University of California, San Francisco.

KYUNG-HEE CHOI, PhD, is a Visiting Postgraduate Scholar at the Center for AIDS Prevention Studies, University of California, San Francisco.

RANI EVERSLEY, PhD, is a Psychologist at the Center for AIDS Prevention Studies, University of California, San Francisco.

PATRICIA FRANKS is a Health Policy Analyst at the Institute for Health Policy Studies and the Center for AIDS Prevention Studies, University of California, San Francisco.

DAVID R. GIBSON, PhD, is an Adjunct Associate Professor, Department of Psychiatry and the Center for AIDS Prevention Studies, University of California, San Francisco; and Senior Research Associate, Haight Ashbury Free Clinics, San Francisco.

EVE GOLDEN, SM, is a Research Associate at the Center for AIDS Prevention Studies, University of California, San Francisco.

JOSEPH R. GUYDISH, PhD, MPH, is a Visiting Postgraduate Scholar at the Center for AIDS Prevention Studies, University of California, San Francisco.

KAREN HEMBRY, PhD, is a Visiting Postgraduate Scholar at the Center for AIDS Prevention Studies, University of California, San Francisco.

JULIE LONDON, PhD, is a Clinical Psychologist and Research Coordinator of Substance Abuse Services at San Francisco General Hospital, Department of Psychiatry, University of California, San Francisco.

JANE LOVELLE-DRACHE, MPH, is a Research Associate in the Department of Psychiatry and the Center for AIDS Prevention Studies, University of California, San Francisco.

EDUARDO S. MORALES, PhD, is a Psychologist in Private Practice and Associate Professor at the California School of Professional Psychology, Alameda.

JOHN L. PETERSON, PhD, is Co-Principal Investigator and Project Director for AIDS Risk Reduction among Black Gay Men at the Center for AIDS Prevention Studies, University of California, San Francisco.

LINDA E. RICO, MPA, is Executive Assistant, Substance Abuse Services at San Francisco General Hospital, Department of Pyschiatry, University of California, San Francisco.

REBECCA L. ROBBINS, MA, is a Research Assistant at the Center for AIDS Prevention Studies, University of California, San Francisco.

JAMES L. SORENSEN, PhD, is an Adjunct Professor and Chief of Substance Abuse Services at San Francisco General Hospital, Department of Psychiatry, University of California, San Francisco.

LAURIE A. WERMUTH, PhD, is an Assistant Professor at the California State University at Chico. (Research for work presented in this volume was conducted while Dr. Wermuth was a faculty member at the University of California, San Francisco.)

Acknowledgments

Many individuals contributed to the material presented in this book. First, we thank the staff and patients of the Substance Abuse Services, San Francisco General Hospital, for their support. Without the support of these people, such a book would not be possible. They participated enthusiastically in both treatment and research efforts, helping to develop improved ways to prevent and treat AIDS among drug abusers. Other drug treatment programs also participated in some of the research projects presented here; we appreciate the participation of those organizations, including the Berkeley Addiction Treatment Services and its director, Walter Byrd; Walden House, Inc., and its director, Alfonso Acampora; and San Francisco's Community Substance Abuse Services and its director, Wayne Clark. We owe a special debt of gratitude to the many individuals who volunteered to participate as subjects in these research studies. Their hard work and willingness to engage in these adventurous activities were essential to the research.

Gratitude is also expressed to our students, colleagues, and assistants in the projects presented here. Many of their names are included in research citations throughout the book. We are especially grateful to Roland Dumontet, Hsiaso-Ti Falcone, Jennifer Ham, Carma Heitzmann, Kenneth Wilkinson, and Mark Young, for the highly significant contributions they made to carrying out these projects.

We also want to extend our appreciation and thanks to the coauthors of specific chapters in this book, who were willing to lend their expertise to this effort.

Our sincere thanks go out to Donald Calsyn, who critiqued the entire book. We are grateful to the coeditor of the Guilford Substance Abuse Series, Thomas R. Kosten, for his initial encouragement, careful scrutiny of the manuscript, and many helpful suggestions. In addition, we thank Seymour Weingarten and Marian Robinson of The Guilford Press, who guided us through the publication and dissemination process.

The research and treatment reported in these pages were supported by a number of sources, including the AIDS Clinical Research Center at the University of California, San Francisco; the city and county of San

Francisco; the University-Wide Task Force on AIDS; and grants from the National Institute on Drug Abuse (Grant Nos. R18DA06097, R18DA06979, R01DA04340, and DA01696) and the National Institute of Mental Health (Grant No. P50MH42459).

Finally, we wish to express our heartfelt appreciation to Linda Rico for the extensive work that went into the editing and preparation of the manuscript.

Although we appreciate the support of those mentioned here, the views and opinions expressed in this book are those of the authors of the individual chapters; they do not reflect the official position or policies of the University of California, San Francisco, or the individuals or organizations whose support we gratefully acknowledge.

Foreword

Injection drug users are the second largest group of persons to have developed AIDS in the United States and in Europe. HIV has also spread widely among injection drug users in South America and in Southeast Asia. Other than in Africa, injection drug users are also the most frequent source of heterosexual and mother–infant transmission of HIV. Reducing the transmission of HIV among and from injection drug users is one of the most formidable problems in the worldwide AIDS epidemic. Research on preventing HIV transmission among and from injection drug users is a relatively new field, dating only from 1981 with the discovery of AIDS among these drug users; it gained the needed technology with the HIV antibody test in 1984, and accelerated with large amounts of U.S. federal and European funding in 1986.

Prior to the discovery of AIDS, there was an extensive research literature on injection drug use, much of which had been conducted in drug abuse treatment programs. Many drug treatment programs have conducted studies of the epidemiology of HIV transmission among injection drug users, but very few have mounted systematic research programs into preventing the transmission of HIV among these drug users. Jim Sorensen and his colleagues in the Substance Abuse Services of the San Francisco General Hospital (SFGH) are a notable exception to this generalization. This book provides a detailed account of their research program. The format of the book is such that it will be extremely useful to staff members in other drug treatment programs who wish to develop AIDS prevention programs for their clients.

There are many reasons why few drug treatment programs have mounted research programs into preventing HIV transmission among injection drug users, and these provide a context for measuring the accomplishments of the SFGH group. First, the amount of federal support for research in this area was not, and generally still is not, adequate to the size of the task. There are, however, other reasons for the paucity of research into preventing HIV transmission in and by this population that are probably more important than the scarcity of research monies (these reasons are discussed in relation to New York City programs in Des Jarlais, 1990).

Many drug treatment programs have denied or attempted to avoid dealing with AIDS among injection drug users. Clients with AIDS have been transferred out of programs, and HIV antibody testing has been used to deny admission to seropositives. AIDS raises a number of difficult issues for drug abuse treatment programs. Although there is no evidence that HIV has ever been transmitted within drug treatment programs, there have been recurrent fears of such transmission. Most drug treatment programs do not have the medical expertise to provide state-of-the-art treatment for HIV-related diseases, and linkages to medical centers that can be expected to have such expertise are relatively rare.

AIDS among clients in a drug treatment program also raises the issues of death and dying. Death rates among injection drug users were high prior to the emergence of AIDS, but treatment programs were relatively isolated from these deaths. The deaths were often sudden (e.g., overdoses or violent deaths), and they typically occurred outside of the drug treatment programs. Treatment staffers rarely had to interact with, much less counsel, a person who had a protracted fatal disease.

Although injection drug users were contracting AIDS as a direct result of their drug use, there are two ways in which AIDS is separate from drug injection that have made it difficult for drug treatment programs to confront AIDS. First, the long latency period between initial HIV infection and the development of AIDS means that one can cease using drugs only to develop AIDS years later. The risks of other fatal consequences of injection drug use essentially become zero after one ceases using the drugs, and this fact is usually incorporated into the counseling of clients. AIDS threatens to undermine the benefits of stopping drug use for clients. For ex-addict staff members, the possibility that they may die from drug use years after stopping their use has been even more distressing.

Second, although HIV infection is strongly associated with injecting illicit drugs, it is not the injection of the drugs themselves that causes the infection, but the microtransfusions that occur when injection equipment is shared. Thus AIDS prevention for injection drug users must address the possibility of "safer" injection—injection of illicit drugs without the sharing of equipment. This has been a very difficult subject for drug abuse treatment program staff members. Prior to the emergence of AIDS, they emphasized to clients the possibility of never again using illicit drugs. Teaching clients about "safer" injections seems to many counselors to undermine the possibility of achieving abstinence from illicit drugs.

Finally, AIDS prevention for injection drug users also needs to include counseling and education about "safer" sex. Prior to the AIDS epidemic, very few drug treatment staff members had ever received any training in human sexuality counseling, and many themselves grew up in social environments that discouraged open and honest communication about sexual issues. Addressing the sexual components of AIDS prevention is not only a task for which staffs have had little or no training, but one that often involves personal embarrassment.

The SFGH substance abuse program has a number of advantages that have helped its staff members to overcome early these obstacles to doing AIDS prevention within a drug abuse treatment setting. Clearly, they are in a city with a high awareness of AIDS and a local culture that is strongly supportive of doing AIDS prevention. They are part of a major medical center that has both state-of-the-art expertise in medical treatment for HIV-related conditions and institutional expertise in obtaining support for prevention and research. The city and state governments have provided funding for both prevention and research. The SFGH group has also had the negative example of New York City, where HIV spread widely among injection drug users prior to awareness of AIDS or any prevention efforts. The rate of HIV exposure among injection drug users in San Francisco was still low at the time the SFGH group began its efforts, so that there was good reason to believe that timely programs could help to prevent most of the problem. Although these geographic and institutional advantages are all important, the most important advantage has been the commitment of the SFGH substance abuse staff to addressing AIDS prevention within a systematic research framework. The level of work that is reflected in this volume comes from the personal commitment of the authors to do something useful about the spread of HIV among injection drug users and their sexual partners.

Much of the information in this volume has been presented at scientific meetings or published in scientific journals. The book, however, provides an opportunity to learn about and understand the prevention work of the SFGH Substance Abuse Services group at a holistic level. Hearing presentations and reading the journal articles are like reading recipes for individual dishes; reading the book is similar to eating a full meal.

In many ways, the AIDS prevention research conducted by the SFGH group is a good model for a research program. An important scientific and practical problem is being addressed, and there is an attempt to address all aspects of the problem. Rigorous methods, such as random assignment to experimental conditions, are used frequently. The research is generally theory-based (the primary theories are the AIDS risk reduction model and the health belief model), so that knowledge can accumulate rapidly. The researchers are also scholars, conceptually integrating their work with that of others in the field. In this book, the use of (disguised) case histories provides a note of personal realism that is often lacking in scientific texts. Finally, the royalties from the book will be donated to the field of AIDS prevention among injection drug users—specifically, to the San Francisco AIDS Foundation for support of its work with Prevention Point, the quasi-legal syringe exchange program in San Francisco.

Don C. Des Jarlais

Preface

The idea for this book came from a conversation between two of its authors. Our research group had been testing out several approaches to slowing the spread of AIDS among drug users and the spread from them to their sexual partners. The studies had much in common: overlapping staff members, measurement instruments, and theoretical orientations. However, we had not yet thought of them as a whole, nor had we considered the implications of what their results would reveal.

The title of this book is meant to express its purpose: to prevent AIDS among drug users and their sexual partners. The book presents the results of several San Francisco experiments aimed at that task. Our research has confirmed our hope that, if drug users receive the right encouragement, they will begin to change in the face of the AIDS epidemic. Targeted AIDS prevention efforts can be effective. Some interventions work, others do not; some policies encourage this change, others are impediments. Although the bulk of the work has taken place in San Francisco, we put this in the context of extensive investigations of other research groups, clinicians, and national and international experts about public policy.

We guide the reader through the topic, beginning with several chapters about AIDS, drug use, sexual behaviors, and theories of change. This is followed by chapters that suggest how to prevent AIDS by action with drug users and their sexual partners. The final part of the book makes concluding recommendations about disseminating prevention programs and forming effective policies. We have covered more topics than normally found in most books that are based on a series of research projects. This is due to the close ties between AIDS research and policy issues, as well as the desire to give more practical, clinical suggestions than would be appropriate for professional journal articles. In addition, the appendix of the book provides resources that can help the reader to get more information or take action. We want to stress the urgency of preventing AIDS in drug users and their sexual partners. As we write, and as readers study this text, the scope of HIV infection continues to widen. Each life lost is a tragedy.

Contents

PART I. AIDS AND DRUG USE

Chapter 1. Introduction: The AIDS–Drug Connection 3
JAMES L. SORENSEN

Chapter 2. Cases: Implications for AIDS Prevention 18
LAURIE A. WERMUTH

Chapter 3. Needle Sharing, Needle Cleaning, and Risk Behavior Change among Injection Drug Users 28
JOSEPH R. GUYDISH, EVE GOLDEN, AND KAREN HEMBRY

Chapter 4. Unsafe Sex and Behavior Change 43
KYUNG-HEE CHOI AND LAURIE A. WERMUTH

Chapter 5. Theoretical Background 62
DAVID R. GIBSON, JOSEPH A. CATANIA, AND JOHN L. PETERSON

PART II. PREVENTIVE INTERVENTIONS WITH DRUG USERS AND THEIR SEXUAL PARTNERS

Chapter 6. Drug Abuse Treatment for HIV-Infected Patients 77
STEVEN L. BATKI AND JULIE LONDON

Chapter 7. Group Counseling to Prevent AIDS 99
JAMES L. SORENSEN, JULIE LONDON, AND EDUARDO S. MORALES

Chapter 8. Individual Counseling 116
DAVID R. GIBSON AND JANE LOVELLE-DRACHE

Chapter 9. Reaching and Counseling Women Sexual Partners 130
LAURIE A. WERMUTH, REBECCA L. ROBBINS, KYUNG-HEE CHOI, AND RANI EVERSLEY

PART III. SOCIAL IMPLICATIONS

Chapter 10. Adopting Effective Interventions 153
JAMES L. SORENSEN AND JOSEPH R. GUYDISH

Chapter 11. Policy Implications 168
LAURIE A. WERMUTH, JAMES L. SORENSEN, AND PATRICIA FRANKS

References 179

Appendix: Where to Get Help or Information 202
LINDA E. RICO

Index 213

Preventing AIDS

in Drug Users and Their Sexual Partners

Part 1

AIDS AND DRUG USE

Chapter 1

Introduction: The AIDS–Drug Connection

JAMES L. SORENSEN

Our first experience with AIDS in our drug treatment population came in 1984, when Victor appeared one morning in the heroin detoxification clinic at San Francisco General Hospital.[1] A Mexican-American in his mid-30s, Victor had come to the program several times before trying to rid himself of a $150-per-day heroin habit, sometimes with temporary success. We had not seen him for a year, and this time he looked different: He had lost nearly 50 pounds and looked worn out. "Victor, you look terrible. What happened to you?" asked the intake worker. He replied matter-of-factly, "Oh, I got AIDS."

Victor died 2 years later. His wife died a year after that. Since the day when Victor came in with AIDS, the drug treatment program at San Francisco General Hospital has changed its admission policies, giving top priority to drug users with symptomatic HIV infection. Through the treatment program, we have attempted to alert other drug users to the threat of AIDS and to contribute to the skills and resolve that they need to avert this disease. We have also developed and evaluated several interventions attempting to slow the spread of AIDS with drug users and their intimate partners. Thus, we write from considerable experience with drug users and AIDS, and we believe that the epidemic can be controlled within this group. This introductory chapter first provides brief descriptions of the medical problems of AIDS, the problems of drug use, the ways in which HIV infection is transmitted, and the current status of AIDS prevention efforts. The second part of the chapter describes the remainder of this book.

AIDS: THE NEW MEDICAL PROBLEM

Acquired immune deficiency syndrome (AIDS) was first recognized as a new clinical syndrome in the United States in 1981. AIDS is sometimes called "HIV disease," because it is caused by the human immunodeficiency virus (HIV), which has been isolated in a variety of human fluids but is most commonly passed between people through blood and semen. Both homosexual and heterosexual activity, as well as injection drug use, play major roles in transmitting HIV infection. Testing for HIV infection has been used for public health and infection control purposes, and also to monitor the epidemic and to identify HIV-infected people who can benefit from early medical intervention.

HIV weakens the immune system. HIV-infected individuals most often progress from latent HIV infection (in which they are basically healthy and identifiable only by laboratory evidence of HIV infection) to having a severely damaged immune system. Along the way they develop a wide range of disease states, from no symptoms to full-blown AIDS. Medical problems with HIV infection range from a mononucleosis-like illness (which can have symptoms similar to drug withdrawal) to chronic lymphadenopathy, night sweats, fever, diarrhea, weight loss, and neuropsychiatric problems (including dementia). A clinical AIDS diagnosis is given to people whose immune systems become unable to protect them against opportunistic infections or cancers that would not develop if their immune systems were intact. The clinical manifestations of HIV infection can involve any of the body's organ systems and can present as dermatological, neurological, pulmonary, gastrointestinal, ophthalmological, or psychiatric problems. As this is written, more than half of the patients diagnosed with AIDS have died, although treatments for the medical problems of AIDS have been developing rapidly.

The wide spectrum of disease states makes AIDS an extremely difficult medical problem. AIDS is creating a large burden on care systems in localities where there are high concentrations of HIV infection. Inpatient care systems can be overrun, and community-based support systems are unable to cope with service demands.

Scientists are racing to develop a vaccine that will neutralize the infectivity of HIV, but they have not yet been successful. HIV displays an unusual degree of genetic variation, which is making development of a vaccine extremely difficult. Researchers are also developing drugs that will kill HIV or slow its replication. To date one drug, zidovudine (AZT), has been clearly demonstrated to slow the progress of HIV infection and is thus an effective treatment. Other drugs are in various stages of development and testing.

In short, AIDS creates a tremendous medical problem. At the present time, the best way to head it off is by lessening the spread of new infections.

AIDS AS A DRUG PROBLEM

People who inject drugs may hold the key to the future of the AIDS epidemic in the United States.[2] As this is written, more than 160,000 people in the United States have been diagnosed with AIDS. The proportion of the people diagnosed with AIDS who are drug users has risen steadily over the years, from slightly over 18% of the 376 cases reported in 1981 (11% heterosexual and 7.1% homosexual or bisexual) to 28.4% of the 43,339 new cases reported in 1990 (23.1% heterosexual and 5.3% homosexual or bisexual), as Table 1.1 illustrates.

TABLE 1.1. Distribution of Reported AIDS Cases (Percentage) by Year of Diagnosis and Exposure Category

Year of diagnosis	Adult IDU[a]	Male homosexual & IDU	Total IDU	Heterosexual	Other[b]
1981	11.0	7.1	(18.1)	0.5	81.4
1982	16.9	9.4	(26.3)	1.1	72.6
1983	17.8	9.4	(26.2)	1.0	71.7
1984	16.7	8.7	(25.4)	1.5	73.1
1985	17.5	7.5	(22.0)	2.0	73.0
1986	18.2	7.8	(26.0)	2.5	71.5
1987	20.1	6.8	(26.9)	3.2	69.9
1988	22.8	6.3	(29.1)	4.1	66.8
1989	23.0	6.3	(29.3)	5.7	65.0
1990[c]	23.1	5.3	(28.4)	6.3	65.3
Total	21.4	6.5	(27.9)	5.2	66.9

Note. Adapted from *AIDS: The Second Decade* (p. 44) by H. G. Miller, C. F. Turner, and L. E. Moses (Eds.), 1990, Washington, DC: National Academy Press. Copyright 1990 by the National Academy of Sciences. Adapted by permission.

[a] Injection drug user.

[b] Includes adult, adolescent, and pediatric cases.

[c] The 1990 figures include only those cases reported through December 31, 1990. All data shown in this table are subject to delays in reporting. Therefore, counts of cases diagnosed in a particular year may understate the number that will ultimately be reported. This type of understatement is particularly likely for cases diagnosed in 1990 and 1991.

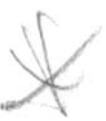

By the last day of 1990, 158,287 adults or adolescents in the United States had been diagnosed with AIDS, of whom 22% had the sole risk factor of intravenous drug use, and another 7% had both injection drug use and another risk factor for HIV infection. AIDS has taken a heavy toll on the poor, urban, and ethnic minority populations in the United States. Furthermore, drug users appear to be the primary link between current high-risk groups and the heterosexual population: The majority of women with AIDS have been injection drug users; in most perinatal cases, the mother or father has a history of injection drug use; a large proportion of male injection drug users appear to have sex partners who do not themselves use drugs, and most heterosexual transmission cases appear to involve sexual contact with an injection drug user. For these reasons, Andrew Moss (1987, p. 389) calls AIDS and injection drug use "the real heterosexual epidemic." We hope that this book will help to alter the epidemic's course.

DRUG USE AND ABUSE

To prevent AIDS, it is important to understand the difficulties that society faces with drug abuse. How extensive is the problem? What drugs are risky for HIV infection? How much does the problem differ across communities or cultural groups? Are the social problems so overwhelming that it does no good to focus on drug use alone? How much are drug users' sexual partners at risk of HIV infection? Specifically, what are the things that put drug users and their sexual partners at risk?

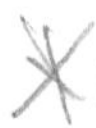

Extent of Drug Use

No one really knows how many injection drug users there are in the United States, and published estimates are not accurate enough to be relied on for forecasting HIV infection among them. There is great variety in injection patterns, which makes it difficult to agree on how to define an "injection drug user." For example, should one count intermittent users? What about a person who uses drugs by injection once per year, once a month, or weekly? Or should we only count those who use a needle every day? In addition, such drug use is generally illegal, making any census of injection drug users subject to undercounting. Several techniques have been used to overcome these problems. Some groups have used indirect estimates based on mathematical models that try to estimate prevalence of drug use from indicators of drug use (e.g., number of drug overdose emergency room admissions); direct estimates based on surveys (e.g., the triannual National Survey on Drug Abuse);

or "informed guesstimates" based on either direct or indirect estimates coupled with personal judgments of experts. A Centers for Disease Control (1987) report that reviewed existing information distinguished between regular drug users, who inject at least once a week, and less frequent users, who inject less often but have used drugs more than just a couple of times. They estimated that there were 900,000 regular users and 200,000 occasional users in 1987, 1.1 million altogether. However, a review of that report indicates that its assumptions are questionable and that a reasonable range is somewhere between 500,000 and 2 million (Spencer, 1989).

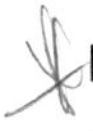

Drugs of Abuse

What drugs are involved in the HIV epidemic? Of the many classes of drugs, opiates and stimulants are the most frequently used drugs that are linked to the risk of HIV infection. Opiates are a class of drugs that have a high potential for abuse; medically, they are used to relieve pain, most frequently in such forms as morphine or Dilaudid. Heroin accounts for 90% of illicit opiate use in the United States and is most frequently used by injection, which is the major route by which drug users transmit HIV. In addition, opiates have immunosuppressant effects, as Chapter 6 explains.

Stimulants are another class of drugs involved in the HIV epidemic. Amphetamines and cocaine are the most common of the stimulants. Amphetamines are most frequently taken in capsules or tablets, but some users may also sniff or inject them. In some regions, such as San Francisco, injectable stimulants ("speed") have been relatively frequently used in the gay community, which has further promoted the spread of HIV. Cocaine (particularly in its smoked form, "crack") has received considerable attention in recent years, both because of a startling increase in its use in the 1980s and because of an indirect association with HIV (explained in Chapter 3). A growing body of research associates cocaine use with HIV problems, including a direct link between injection cocaine use and HIV prevalence rates, and associations between crack use and sexual risk behaviors.

Central nervous system depressants have been directly linked with the HIV epidemic because of their strong association with sexual behaviors that transmit HIV. Depressants, such as the related sedative-hypnotics (commonly called sleeping pills and tranquilizers), can have disinhibiting effects on behavior at low doses, and several studies have found that among gay men and heterosexual couples, alcohol use and unsafe sex go together. (Alcohol is also a central nervous system depressant.) Chapter 3 explains more about this issue.

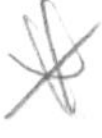

Hallucinogens or psychedelics have not been closely linked with the HIV epidemic. They create profound changes in mood and perceptions. Their use does not commonly involve needle use. Like depressants, they can create disinhibiting effects. In theory, these could cause people to be more likely to have unsafe sex, but we are not aware of studies that have demonstrated a strong link between hallucinogen use and HIV risk.

Regional Variation

There is considerable regional variation in injection drug abuse. In general, it is more common in urban areas. For example, a May 1990 report from the U.S. Senate showed the number of "hard-core" (weekly or more) cocaine users to vary from 1.1 per 1,000 population in South Dakota to 24.4 per 1,000 population in New York (U.S. Senate Committee on the Judiciary, 1990).

Likewise, HIV infection and AIDS are not spread evenly across communities. Instead, the largest concentrations of AIDS cases per population have been found in the District of Columbia, New York, California, New Jersey, and Florida; the largest concentrations of HIV infection among military recruits have been found in the District of Columbia, Puerto Rico, New York, Maryland, and New Jersey (Centers for Disease Control, 1987). The prevalence of HIV infection among injection drug users shows considerable variation, ranging from 50 to 60% in urban northern New Jersey, Puerto Rico, and New York City, to less than 5% in many states in the central and western parts of the country. There is some encouragement in these differences: As we learn how to prevent the spread of HIV infection, these lessons can be applied to drug users in communities that have not yet suffered widespread exposure to the virus. However, AIDS cases are appearing more frequently in areas that were previously spared from the epidemic (Miller, Turner, & Moses, 1990).

Ethnic and Cultural Issues

There is considerable cultural diversity among drug users, and it is important to understand the cultural and ethnic variations that are so integral to this disease. First, there is variation in prevalence of AIDS: Although African-Americans make up only 12% of the national population, about 28% of AIDS cases in adults and 52% of the pediatric cases have been among African-Americans. Hispanics also are overrepresented in AIDS cases. Although 6% of the general population is Hispanic, about 16% of AIDS cases in adults and 26% of pediatric cases have been among Hispanics. Also, numerous studies have shown the HIV infection rates among African-American and Hispanic drug users to be higher than among whites. In addition, there are differences among cultures in the prevalent injecting practices, in the use of "shooting galleries" (places where drug users congregate to inject drugs), and in friendship patterns; these differences make it important to develop enough prevention techniques that some will be effective with the wide band of cultural groups involved with the injection of drugs. The issues of ethnicity and culture are so important that we have attempted to comment on these in each chapter of the book.

Ties to Social Problems

The drug users and women at highest risk for AIDS are culturally disadvantaged, with few economic or educational resources. These factors make it doubly difficult to build the self-confidence and skills needed to avoid HIV infection. Some groups have been critical of programs that try to apply inexpensive solutions, such as bleach distribution or needle exchanges; these critics contend that such programs are giving the poor a sop rather than offering real help, which is more expensive. Others point out that AIDS prevention programs already have monumental tasks and must do what they can; they cannot be asked to eliminate poverty as well.

Sexual Partners of Drug Users

Table 1.1 shows that the proportion of U.S. adult/adolescent AIDS cases resulting from heterosexual transmission has risen from 0.5% in 1981 to 5.2% in 1990. Among women, the statistics are much more dramatic: 34% of the AIDS cases diagnosed among women in 1990 resulted from heterosexual transmission. Much of this spread comes from drug-injecting men. Unfortunately, few preventive programs have been implemented with these women, and even fewer have been demonstrated to be effective.

LEVELS OF DEFENSE AGAINST HIV INFECTION

What are the activities that put drug users and their sexual partners at risk for HIV infection? Among injection drug users and their sexual partners, the behaviors that lead to HIV infection fall into two major categories, drug use and sexual practices. When we conduct AIDS prevention activities, our approach is to emphasize a hierarchical structure of defense lines against HIV infection, as shown in Figure 1.1. The defense lines at the perimeters of the circles are the most desirable, and defenses become increasingly risky as one approaches the centers of the circles. This "levels of defense" model of AIDS prevention suggests that multiple programs and policies at each level of defense can slow the spread of AIDS.

Drug Use

In regard to drug use, abstinence provides the strongest line of defense against AIDS, as Figure 1.1 depicts. When they are "loaded," people are more likely to engage in a variety of risky activities. To prevent HIV infection at this level, programs should emphasize prevention of the initiation into drug use; alcohol and drug education; treatment programs for injection drug users that enable them to give up their drug use; and relapse prevention activities that enable them to continue abstinence. Community efforts to prevent youths from advancing to drug use may ultimately have an important preventive effect.

For those who continue to use drugs, Figure 1.1 shows that a less perfect defense is not to use needles. Interventions can be implemented to prevent the progression to needle use. For example, Des Jarlais and colleagues organized a group-oriented program for adolescents who were "sniffing" drugs, aiming to discourage the progression to needle use (Des Jarlais, Friedman, Casriel, & Kott, 1987a). This level of defense can also involve identifying high-risk groups for intervention, delivering culturally appropriate educational information to them, and fostering peer support for safer practices.

For those who continue to use needles, not sharing needles will help to slow the progression of HIV. Although "don't share needles" is a simple message, it is shorthand for several elements of drug paraphernalia that may be contaminated and yield infection. The syringe, needle, "cooker" (small container used to dissolve the injectable drug), "cotton" (used to strain out impurities from the solution in the cooker), and rinse water (used to rinse out syringes and needles before they are reused) can all pass HIV from one drug user to another. Preventive programs at this level of defense can provide education about HIV infection to injection drug users, with the idea that they will decide not to share, or at least to cut down on the number of people with whom they do share needles. Needle distribution and exchange schemes also come into play here: A major reason that drug users give for continuing to share is the lack of available clean needles, and exchange programs can reduce that reason for sharing. In addition, there are technological advances in process to develop and market "single-use" syringes that

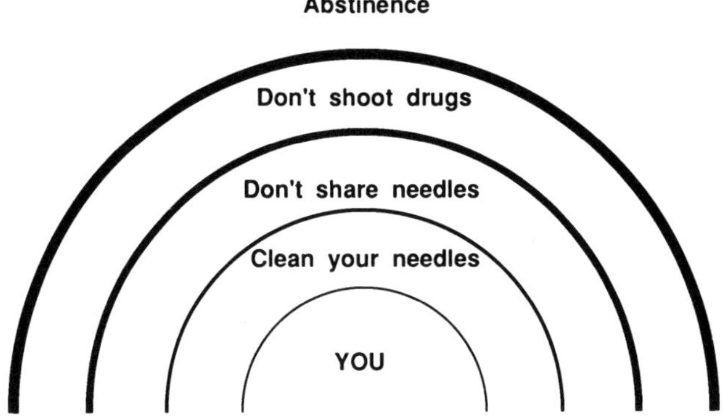

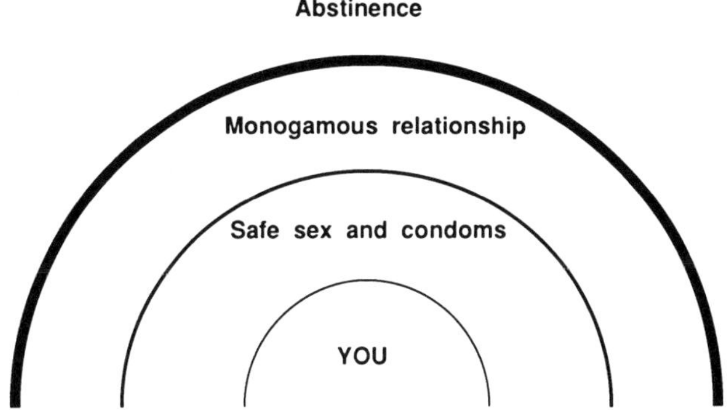

FIGURE 1.1. Defenses against AIDS: Drug use and sexual activity. From "Community Drug Use and AIDS" by J. L. Sorensen, C. Heitzmann, and J. R Guydish, 1990, *Journal of Clinical Psychology, 18,* p. 350. Copyright 1990 by the Clinical Psychology Publishing Company. Reprinted by permission.

will make it impossible to reuse a syringe. Providing HIV antibody testing to injection drug users can also be thought of at this level, with the idea that special treatment programs may encourage the HIV-infected drug users to move to a higher-level defense against spreading HIV, both by educating them about the dangers that they pose for others and by providing drug and AIDS treatment specifically for them.

For those who do share needles, Figure 1.1 shows that a last line of defense is to "clean" (sterilize) them each time between users. Programs can educate drug users about needle-cleaning techniques and even distribute small vials of alcohol or bleach, along with new cookers and cottons, in a last-ditch effort to help them avoid HIV infection.

Sexual Activities

Abstinence is also the best defense against acquiring AIDS through sexual activity, as the lower half of Figure 1.1 shows. Family influence and school education programs can help people to delay sexual activity, and educational programs for people at risk can help them to emphasize this level of defense. Programs that tout abstinence only, however, have limited appeal and practicality. As one woman said at one of our AIDS prevention workshops, "The only way I can ever have a family is to have what you call 'unsafe sex.'" With adults, it is difficult to promote abstinence from sexual activities.

For people who are not abstinent, a mutually monogamous relationship (with an uninfected partner who does not inject drugs) may be the next most effective defense. Suggestions to choose sexual partners carefully, sometimes with mutual HIV antibody testing, can also be viewed at this level of defense. It is important to note, however, that if a drug user is engaging in risky needle use, then even a monogamous sexual relationship provides no protection for the sexual partner: A drug user can acquire HIV through the needle and pass it on to a partner through sexual activity. As Chapter 9 explains, many women perceive their AIDS risk in terms of the drug use behavior of their partners. For them, mutual sexual monogamy provides only a thin veneer of safety. In fact, their sexual relationship may be riskier than if they had several sexual partners who did not inject drugs.

The last line of defense against contracting AIDS through sexual activity, as Figure 1.1 shows, is to engage only in "safe" sexual practices. Usually this refers to using barrier methods, such as condoms, to prevent HIV-infected body fluids from entering the sexual partner's body. Prevention programs can educate injection drug users and their sexual partners about the importance and the mechanics of safe sexual practices, and they can distribute items such as condoms and spermicides.

INITIAL STEPS IN PREVENTION

Early in the AIDS epidemic, there were several years in which HIV infection statistics steadily grew among drug users. For example, in New York, the virus entered the drug-using group during the mid-1970s and spread rapidly in 1979 through 1983. From 1984 through

1987, however, seroprevalence rates stabilized at between 55% and 60% among injection drug users applying to treatment programs. A similar time course was seen in San Francisco, with studies of HIV seroprevalence showing 3–5% in 1984, rapidly growing to 12–16%, and then leveling off. The stabilization of seroprevalence should not be confused with eliminating the transmission of HIV: Cohort studies continue to show new infections occurring each year. Likewise, the proportion of AIDS cases who are drug users increased for many years, but in 1988, 1989, and 1990 drug users comprised a steady 29% of the new cases (see Table 1.1).

It is clear that drug users can and will change their risk behaviors. In San Francisco, studies have shown startling increases in drug users' use of bleach to clean needles, and large decreases in self-reported needle sharing among injection drug users applying to treatment programs. These changes have occurred in a community that is implementing interventions at all levels of defense against AIDS. Outreach workers have given information and taught about bleach on the streets and in the shooting galleries. Programs have conducted outreach in mobile vans. Education programs have been developed and implemented in treatment programs. HIV antibody testing has been made widely available, with high-quality counseling about the meaning of the results. Special drug abuse treatment slots have been designated for people with AIDS. An underground needle exchange collects used syringes and replaces them with clean ones. An array of written materials, videos, and public service announcements has spread the word about AIDS. However, the wider-reaching, more expensive social changes have still not occurred. There are still waiting lists to get into drug treatment programs, and not enough outreach workers to educate the people who are at risk.

HOW TO USE THIS BOOK

In this book, we aim to disseminate research-validated information about how to prevent HIV infection among drug users and their sexual partners. The book is for practitioners and scientists coping with the problems of drug abuse and AIDS, and for those involved in the search for AIDS prevention techniques with other population groups such as adolescents. It comes from our experience in developing and evaluating AIDS prevention programs with drug abusers and their sexual partners.

The health professionals who work with drug users have many questions about what they can do to slow the spread of HIV infection among their patients and their patients' intimate partners and children.

They may be discouraged by the denial of risk for HIV infection in these groups and their own inability to get drug users to change behaviors. They want to know, to put it simply, what works. What can they do to prevent the spread of AIDS in their clinics, in their professional practices, or among friends who may be risking HIV infection by having unsafe sexual encounters? The book addresses these issues.

Organization

Eleven chapters are organized into three sections covering the following broad topics: (1) problems of drug abuse and AIDS; (2) interventions with drug users and their sexual partners; and (3) conclusions and policy recommendations.

In Chapter 2, Laurie Wermuth presents several individual case examples that illustrate some of the problems faced by injection drug users and their sexual partners. The stories of these people illustrate how individuals, local resources, and social policies connect to make it more or less likely that HIV infection will spread. The cases make the point that positive steps can be taken to arrest the expansion of HIV infection and AIDS among these populations.

In Chapter 3, Joseph Guydish, Eve Golden, and Karen Hembry explain the extent to which needle use puts drug users at risk, as well as ways in which the risks can be lowered. They emphasize how important it is to understand the social context of injection drug use before attempting to prevent HIV among drug users. Their review documents how many changes have taken place in needle sharing and needle cleaning, giving special attention to New York and San Francisco, where several studies have occurred. They also provide an overview of the AIDS prevention interventions that have been attempted with injection drug users, and comment on the future directions of interventions to prevent the spread of HIV through needle use.

In Chapter 4, Kyung-Hee Choi and Laurie Wermuth emphasize that drug users and their sexual partners risk transmitting HIV through their sexual behaviors. They describe sexual behaviors that are risky for transmitting HIV, as well as the difficulties associated with behavioral changes among injection drug users and their sexual partners. In describing AIDS risk behaviors, they critically examine what is known about the risk to sexual partners, the risks of sexual practices, and perceptions of AIDS risk. They extend these issues to the difficulties associated with changing risky sexual behaviors, presenting data that have not been reported before. They give special attention to the extent of condom use and factors influencing the use of condoms, with the aim of providing the groundwork for future research.

In Chapter 5, David Gibson, Joseph Catania, and John Peterson explain concepts and theories that have helped in understanding why these risky behaviors are so intractable and how interventions can attempt to change them. They emphasize the use of a new model for understanding risk reduction, the AIDS risk reduction model, which they explain in detail. They also examine the predictive ability of theories emphasizing ecological and social factors. The chapter presents several new analyses of previously unreported data, to provide a better understanding of how robustly these theories can predict actual risk behaviors of drug users.

Altogether, the intent of these first five chapters is to educate readers about drug abuse and AIDS problems, rather than their solutions. Chapters 6 through 9 comprise the section on how readers can encourage drug abusers and their sexual partners to change. This is not a "how to" manual, but a research-oriented text; nevertheless, these chapters contain a number of practical suggestions that should be useful to health professionals, friends, and concerned family members.

In Chapter 6, Steven Batki and Julie London review drug abuse treatment as an intervention with drug abusers, giving special attention to drug abusers who have already been infected with HIV. They discuss how treatment of drug abuse is AIDS prevention in and of itself, and they review the types of drug treatment programs that are commonly available in the United States. They also present a care model for providing mental health services to HIV-infected drug users, and provide several suggestions for future research and treatment.

In Chapter 7, Julie London, Eduardo Morales, and I review research information about a group education approach and ways to apply it in different drug treatment settings. We explain the variety of group counseling approaches that are being developed to prevent AIDS, as well as the evidence of impact for these interventions. We also describe, in some detail, how such groups have worked with drug abusers in San Francisco treatment programs. In addition, we make suggestions for future development of the group approach.

In Chapter 8, David Gibson and Jane Lovelle-Drache describe individual counseling about AIDS risks for individuals with drug problems. Their intervention is based on the AIDS risk reduction model and involves 65–75 minutes of counseling, and they explain how the counseling is conducted.

In Chapter 9, Laurie Wermuth, Rebecca Robbins, Kyung-Hee Choi, and Rani Eversley discuss the risks faced by women sexual partners of injection drug users and review issues pertinent to preventive intervention. They point out that the percentage of female AIDS cases attributable to heterosexual transmission is continuing to rise, and that much of this heterosexual spread comes from drug-injecting men. They review the literature about women, AIDS risks, and the constraints on self-protection. They suggest that preventive actions are needed on several levels, including the mass media, medical clinics, drug treatment clinics, and special AIDS prevention projects for women and for heterosexual men. They also describe, in some detail, a project to counsel women at risk in the San Francisco Bay Area, and they discuss their women clients' HIV prevention strategies and clinical issues. They point out that individual counseling, although advantageous in some ways, is very limited in its likely effect on women's sexual partners, and they suggest several directions for future program development and research.

Chapters 10 and 11 present conclusions and recommendations for developing policy. In Chapter 10, Joseph Guydish and I discuss the application of technology: how to get effective prevention projects into the field. We suggest that people contemplating interventions should base them on an understanding of why drug users and sexual partners do things that are risky for AIDS transmission. We provide specific guidelines for assessing the evidence that purported prevention projects are effective, pointing out the common limitations in the existing evaluations of interventions. Finally, we suggest several principles for distributing interventions, based on the lessons of dissemination/utilization research.

In Chapter 11, the final chapter, Laurie Wermuth and I make suggestions for policy-oriented activities in prevention, research, and treatment of AIDS among drug users and their sexual partners. This chapter and the book conclude by emphasizing that solutions to the problems of AIDS will need to come from within the affected cultural groups to be effective, but that policy makers can promote this needed mobilization.

Suggestions to Readers

Each reader will use this book differently. To understand the ingredients needed to prevent AIDS among drug abusers or their sexual partners, we recommend that readers begin with Part I. For readers who are particularly interested in preventing AIDS, Part II (Chapters 6–9) may be most useful. If readers have questions concerning how to do these activities, the Appendix provides a resource guide. Part III will be most useful for the policy makers or health program planners who need to make tough, creative decisions about how to shape care systems.

It is in the best interest of most health professionals to learn as much as they can about drug abuse and AIDS. People who have a problem with drugs are in need of health care professionals who understand. They need an ally in their efforts to change, and their most effective allies can be informed health care professionals. Such professionals can be very helpful in providing compassionate care, and program developers need to be familiar with these problems to design effective prevention programs. Ultimately, it will be in the best interest of future generations to assist drug abusers and their sexual partners in putting a stop to the AIDS epidemic. By helping to stop HIV transmission now, health professionals and community members will be saving future generations from the devastating health problems of AIDS.

NOTES

[1]This book has considerable case material. In describing situations that reflect real lives, we have altered, eliminated, and disguised information that might identify individuals, and have disassociated sensitive material from them. Put simply, beauticians have become plumbers, uncles have become cousins, and so forth; in similar fashion, we have changed locations, sexes, ages, and so on, but in ways that do not alter the meaning of the cases.

[2]This book refers to people who self-administer drugs via hypodermic needle as "injection" drug users rather than "intravenous" drug users, because the former term encompasses those who inject drugs into muscles or under the skin rather than solely into veins. Such injection is assumed to be risky for transmission of HIV. Using an operational definition, we have also distinguished between "users" and "abusers" of drugs: Presence in a drug treatment program signals that a person's drug use has become problematic abuse. Finally, the text uses "African-American" rather than "black" as an ethnicity description, except where the population referred to is primarily from the Caribbean.

Chapter 2

Cases: Implications for AIDS Prevention

LAURIE A. WERMUTH

> Some have seen the AIDS epidemic in a purely "moral" light: AIDS is a disease that occurs among those who violate the moral order. As one journalist concluded: "Suddenly a lot of people fear that they and their families might suddenly catch some mysterious, fatal illness which until now has been confined to society's social outcasts." AIDS, like other sexually transmitted diseases, has been viewed as a fateful link between social deviance and the morally correct.
>
> —Allan M. Brandt (1988, p. 155)

With the AIDS epidemic has come greater awareness of the invisible world of injection drug use, but not necessarily greater understanding of the inhabitants of that world. Even those who have worked closely with drug-dependent individuals often remain awestruck by the powers of addiction. The spread of HIV infection has added new risks to the already dangerous careers of injection drug users, and new challenges to drug treatment programs. In this chapter, case examples illustrate some of the problems faced by drug injectors and their sexual partners. Their responses to those problems and the potential for positive action are tied closely to the likelihood that these groups will slow the spread of HIV infection.

PEARL: A LITTLE STIMULUS AND A LOT OF RESPONSE

This story is extraordinary in that one person did so many constructive things for herself and others. The case is described and then discussed in terms of the strategies Pearl brought to bear on her situation and the positive influences that shaped her responses. Pearl's case is atypical, yet it sheds light on what is possible in HIV prevention. Her case gives us clues as to how we can help catalyze such endeavors through programs and policies.

Pearl is an African-American woman in her early 30s, married with four children. She has had a long-term codeine dependency, and she had occasionally injected drugs with her husband. She first used codeine as an adolescent when her doctor prescribed it for pain. It subsequently became her "drug of choice" for self-medicating emotional and physical discomfort.

Pearl had heard and read news stories about drug users and AIDS before she was interviewed and individually counseled by a research project for sexual partners of men who injected drugs. She had also attended a group session on HIV prevention at her drug treatment clinic. She was disturbed about what she saw in her husband (who still injected cocaine and heroin), in his friends, and in her neighborhood. Her husband was not using sterilized needles, and there were people in her neighborhood who seemed to be dying of AIDS without receiving regular medical care. She described others who were injecting drugs and having sex without taking the needed precautions to keep the AIDS virus from spreading.

These influences had motivated Pearl to do something about the conditions around her. Group and individual counseling (in the clinic and the research project) provided forums in which to express her thoughts, get support, and obtain supplies such as condoms and small bleach bottles, to distribute to her husband and around her neighborhood. Pearl also became the enforcer in her own home, setting down the rule that "Shooting up is not allowed here" and posting it for acquaintances to see. Since she could not stop her husband from using drugs, Pearl supplied him with bleach for cleaning his needles, and she insisted they always use condoms when having sex. Her husband complied with her wishes at first, although it was a struggle at times. She had a sprained wrist at her follow-up research interview 3 months later—an injury she had sustained in a fight with her husband over her rule of no drugs in the home. Although this was discouraging, Pearl had not lost her resolve. Her husband had again promised to adhere to their agreements about not using drugs at home and about using condoms.

Pearl's case cautions us to be wary of stereotypes, particularly those of the drug abuser incapacitated against the AIDS epidemic. Although the population of drug injectors is vastly different from mobilized groups of gay men in terms of the resources they can bring to bear in protecting themselves from HIV, it is possible for individuals to take action and bring about results. Pearl had suffered a beating by her husband; however, she neither felt herself to be a passive victim nor behaved as one. Their relationship seemed to be a fairly egalitarian one, in which both members participated in decisions about child rearing, home environment, and money. It annoyed her husband when Pearl pressured him to stop using drugs and to keep them out of the house, but he did not question her right to raise those issues.

Many threads make up Pearl's experience. Several factors enabled this woman to turn motivation into positive choices and actions. Although her story seems uniquely individual, her actions were influenced by cultural and institutional contexts.

First, the mass media played a role in Pearl's education about AIDS, sensitizing her to the problem and alerting her to the danger of AIDS. She had heard stories on television and radio and read articles in newspapers that had raised her interest and caused her worry.

The drug treatment program that Pearl attended had an excellent group counseling format, which featured a variety of educational presentations, including those on HIV prevention. The waiting room had posters and brochures containing prevention information. Pearl participated in a research project made available through the clinic. She was interviewed and given individual HIV prevention counseling. The interview and counseling did not change Pearl, but contributed to her awareness, gave her support, and provided some basic resources that facilitated actions she was already eager to take.

In addition, Pearl's friends and acquaintances were valuable in sharing information. She saw these people frequently, and many of them were connected by ties of family, work, and social life. Several writers have noted the importance of networks in AIDS prevention (e.g., Friedman et al., 1990; Valdiserri, 1989). Valdiserri writes about networks within minority communities, "If we have access to a social structure that can not only transmit information about AIDS prevention but that also has the capability to endorse such information as valuable and consequential to its members, we have a potent means of introducing normative change" (pp. 119–120). Friedman and his colleagues (1990) stress the value of providing assistance to enhance indigenous networks in mobilizing their own AIDS prevention efforts.

The city in which this program was located also shaped Pearl's response. For example, there was an absence of draconian policies calling for the arrest of individuals carrying bleach bottles (as drug use paraphernalia), as well as an absence of harassment in her poor, largely African-American neighborhood. If the police had maintained a repressive profile in her city, Pearl might never have considered doing her outreach work. On the negative side, the city lacked outreach and prevention activities in high-risk neighborhoods. Had a needle exchange program and outreach activities been available, not as many individuals would have been at risk because of contaminated needles, and Pearl could have referred her acquaintances to those services.

Pearl's case also highlights the personal process of coming to grips with HIV risk. For some this comes slowly and is hindered by denial and other obstacles; for Pearl it came quickly, and her fear of AIDS was swiftly turned to positive action. A twofold lesson for those who counsel individuals emerges from Pearl's story: We must be clear and forceful in our presentation of the realities of risk, yet at the same time must help individuals devise strategies and solutions that are realistic and positive. We can expect the best while being prepared and supportive in working with the most difficult of problems.

Pearl's case provides several lessons on policy and practice in HIV prevention:

1. Individuals can be mobilized to take action in their communities with institutional support and resources.
2. Within families and couples, individuals can be instrumental in establishing preventive practices.
3. The social networks of individuals who inject drugs, linked by acquaintance, exchange networks, and family ties, can be effective in quickly spreading information, and eventually in changing the norms of drug use and sexual practices.
4. The print and broadcast media, videos, and brochures play an important role in gaining the attention of those who are unaware of their own danger of acquiring HIV infection.
5. Drug treatment clinics play a central role in educating and promoting changes in drug use and sexual norms, and in individually counseling clients about their risk.
6. Research projects that intervene can act as catalysts, especially among those already concerned and motivated to take constructive actions.
7. Local governments can promote HIV prevention through outreach activities staffed by paid and volunteer workers, as well as through the absence of punitive policies.

MARTY: SAFE NEEDLES, UNSAFE SEX

The man we discuss in this second example highlights a pattern that often frustrates drug treatment and AIDS prevention counselors. The case description is followed by a discussion of the denial of sexual risk taking, as well as influences affecting injection drug users' recognition of that risk. Marty's statements reveal several of a wide range of defensive responses to the threat of AIDS: Some of these bring about positive actions, and others block preventive changes and induce anxiety.

Marty is a white man in his mid-40s who had ceased to inject drugs and was enrolled in a methadone maintenance program. He discussed his experiences when attending a voluntary group session about AIDS at his clinic. Marty felt good about encouraging his friends to be careful. He enthusiastically described teaching his acquaintances how to use bleach properly to sterilize their drug-injecting equipment, and he continued to take small bottles of bleach to them. At a later point in the discussion, Marty revealed that he was afraid to get tested for the HIV antibody because he had shared needles with someone who later became sick with symptoms of HIV infection. He explained that he doubted that he could cope with a positive result. Another client asked Marty whether he was having sex, and he replied that there were several women with whom he regularly had sex. When asked by the counselor who was facilitating the discussion whether he used condoms, he replied, "No, because I just don't think I have [HIV]."

Marty's contribution to AIDS prevention in the area of needle practices was not matched by attention to his own sexual behavior. What was disturbing—and frustrating to the counselor who was trying to help—was that Marty seemed unaware of his contradictory behaviors. Perhaps the threat of spreading the AIDS virus through sex seemed a less immediate danger.

Marty's denial about his possible HIV infection resulted in his putting his sexual partners at risk. It is important for AIDS prevention counselors and drug treatment counselors to recognize and address this splitting of behaviors and rationales. It is important for policy makers and the public to understand that this phenomenon is not unique to drug users, but is a common one among individuals faced with dangers in their everyday lives. These psychological processes are an important element that must be recognized in effective counseling, whether it occurs in conjunction with HIV antibody testing, drug treatment, or medical care, or in the course of outreach work.

Participation in a drug treatment program allowed Marty to stop injecting drugs and to have a relatively stable lifestyle. It also gave him the presence of mind to be aware and concerned about AIDS risk among others. As Chapter 6 discusses in detail, the drug treatment program played a positive role in addition to providing treatment. For example, information about correct cleaning procedures and access to small bleach bottles made it possible for Marty to become an AIDS educator, reaching individuals who did not attend clinics or have contact with outreach workers. In attending the group, Marty received positive support for his AIDS outreach activities and also was confronted regarding his unsafe sexual practices. Clinic counselors also addressed HIV prevention issues with all clients in individual counseling sessions.

Brochures, posters, and video presentations provided constant reminders of AIDS, and group sessions gave clients opportunities to discuss the problem together. We do not know whether Marty began to use condoms or have fewer sexual partners, but we do know that his group session brought the issue to his attention among his peers. The issue was to be pursued in his individual counseling, so we can hope that positive and consistent persuasion helped to bring about change.

Marty's case provides an opportunity to address the broader social response to AIDS. We may react with frustration to Marty's practice of unprotected sex. Yet his apparent disregard may reflect a more general social reluctance to acknowledge the heterosexual spread of HIV. Although scientific evidence of transmission of HIV by vaginal intercourse has existed since the early years of the epidemic, only recently has this mode of transmission been given much attention. Perhaps in part because the cases of full-blown AIDS were slow to accumulate among heterosexuals in the United States, the issue was not pursued as forcefully or visibly as was the connection between anal intercourse and AIDS among gay men, or needle practices and AIDS among drug users. Unlike the formulation for African countries, HIV transmission here was conceived of as largely confined to the stigmatized groups of gay men and drug addicts, and a few "innocent victims" (Brandt, 1988; Treichler, 1988). Within this ideological context, the morally deviant practice of drug injecting (Ben Yehuda, 1990) coincided with its greater efficiency in transmitting the virus, thus enabling quiescence regarding sexual transmission.

The neglect of heterosexual transmission has had the harshest consequences for infected women and the infants born to them. Only relatively recently has alarm registered as the numbers of women diagnosed with AIDS (according to Centers for Disease Control criteria) have increased and the numbers of infected infants have risen. AIDS has become the leading cause of death among young African-American women in the states of New Jersey and New York, and is approaching ranking fifth in the causes of death among all women in the United States (Coleman, 1990). Many women who inject drugs are doubly at risk through the sharing of needles, if only with their one male partner, and sexual intercourse. Once diagnosed with AIDS, women die far more quickly than do gay men. Moreover, the epidemiological evidence does not support the characterization of women in the sex industry as "vectors of disease," but rather suggests that resistance to condom use among heterosexual men who engage in risk behaviors is a key obstacle in the fight against AIDS.

In sum, Marty's case highlights three implications for practice and policy:

1. The clinical challenge in addressing individuals' denial about contradictory behaviors and in confronting the rationalizations used to explain them.
2. The role of drug treatment programs in promoting safer behavior.
3. Public neglect, until recently, of the heterosexual transmission of HIV in the United States.

JAN AND BILL: MIDDLE-CLASS CONFIDENCE ERODED BY THE STIGMA OF AIDS AND ADDICTION

Jan and Bill are a middle-class white couple in their mid-20s who had injected drugs for a few years. Jan worked full-time in a record store, and Bill worked sporadically in restaurants. Jan had stopped injecting drugs several times and had attempted unsuccessfully to persuade Bill to do the same. In an attempt to get them both to stop together (and to prevent her own relapse), Jan arranged for them to move to the country, away from their drug-using friends. A few months later, however, they moved back. Neither Bill nor Jan wished to receive long-term drug treatment, although they had received medications for withdrawal symptoms from a detoxification clinic.

The AIDS epidemic shocked Jan out of complacency about their drug use, but it did not affect Bill's attitudes. Jan described two incidents that shocked and frightened her. The first occurred when she discovered a stash of used needles that Bill had brought home. When she asked him about the needles, he explained that someone had given them to him and he brought them home, "just in case they ran out of new ones." Since they had always had a supply of new needles (from a friend who was a nurse), and they didn't share needles with others outside their relationship, Jan had not worried about AIDS before. Finding the used needles suddenly made her realize that Bill could have been sharing needles with others and might have been infected. She realized that he could pass the virus to her.

The second incident occurred when Jan was having intestinal problems and needed minor skin surgery. She went to several doctors, and at each visit, the nurses were pleasant until she rolled up her sleeve to have her blood pressure checked. The nurses then excused themselves to speak with the doctor. In each case they returned to say that they would not be able to help her. Jan's scars from needle use caused her to be refused medical care. As Jan told the interviewer, she was horrified: "I had never been treated like a drug addict before. They must have thought I had AIDS or something."

We include this case as a reminder that some individuals who inject drugs do not match the general profile of injection drug users. Thus far, this couple had avoided trouble with the law, had escaped serious medical problems, had not stolen to support their habits, and had a supply of sterile needles. Jan not only was upset that she was refused medical care, but also was shocked that individuals whom she considered her social equals treated her as a stigmatized addict. Coming as she did from an upper-middle-class background (and a family ignorant of her drug use), she had never been treated this way. It came to her as a painful reminder that others regarded the drug injecting that she had made a normal part of her life as highly deviant. It also shocked her into realizing she could be infected with HIV.

"Closeted" drug injectors such as Jan and Bill are often not in contact with drug treatment clinics or outreach workers. They can be alerted to the AIDS epidemic by the media, brochures, educational programs through medical clinics, places of employment, schools, and acquaintances. Individuals in these circumstances can be assisted by clear messages through a variety of channels, as well as access to anonymous HIV antibody testing, counseling, needle exchange, and condom promotion programs. However, not all drug users are so responsive, as the next vignette illustrates.

ALFRED: HIV DISEASE AND DRUG TREATMENT

Alfred's case is presented to illustrate some of the needs of the HIV-symptomatic drug treatment client, as well as the challenge to (and tremendous burden on) drug treatment clinics to meet those needs.

Alfred walked into the methadone detoxification clinic at San Francisco General Hospital, tired and ready to take a break from his running after heroin and cocaine. He had lost a great deal of weight and had an oral thrush infection. The intake nurse gave him an examination and informed him that although these symptoms could be a result of his weakened physical condition, they could also be symptoms of HIV infection. The nurse asked whether he wished to take an HIV antibody test, and he agreed. When the test came back positive, and Alfred was counseled about the infection, its modes of transmission, and his drug treatment options. Alfred was placed on a steady, maintenance-level dose of methadone.

The intake nurse made arrangements for Alfred concurrently to attend the HIV outpatient clinic in the adjacent building. He also asked about Alfred's living circumstances and made phone calls to locate temporary housing. The counselor then asked about his sex life: Had he had sex recently? If so, he should let those individuals know that they might have been exposed to the virus and that they might want to get tested. Alfred hadn't had sex recently, but he said he would think back to the last times and consider talking to those people.

By the time Alfred transferred to the maintenance clinic, he was feeling a bit stronger. He had stopped injecting drugs, but he still snorted cocaine occasionally. Alfred's counselor laid out his treatment plan: He was to see her every day for counseling, and he would also see the doctor or nurse when he felt ill. His counselor offered to help keep track of his appointments with the HIV clinic, and to assist him with other problems he might encounter. The doctor and counselor confronted Alfred on his continued cocaine use, reminding him that it was a breach of clinic rules as well as hazardous to his already precarious health.

After a month in the maintenance program, problems began to emerge that called for special solutions. Alfred was hospitalized periodically; symptoms of dementia began to appear; he occasionally missed attending the clinic; and tests of urine samples revealed continued cocaine use. The clinic had procedures in place to accommodate HIV-affected clients that had been worked out during prior experience with such clients. A "low-threshold" treatment protocol had been developed to maximize the HIV-infected individuals' ability to remain in the program.

The medical director consulted with Alfred's physicians in the HIV ward regarding his dementia and other symptoms, and his counselor requested referrals to volunteers that might help Alfred get to his clinic appointments. Alfred's urine samples were tested weekly so that his counselor could continue to closely monitor and confront his cocaine abuses.

Several levels of care can be provided within drug treatment programs for the problems of HIV-infected patients. These include help with material supports (such as housing, welfare funds, meals, transportation, and health care), education about HIV, self-help groups, supportive psychotherapy, and (when needed) the use of psychiatric medications. In addition, a concerted effort should be made to reach and counsel the sexual partners of infected clients.

Alfred's case illustrates the need for flexibility, intensive counseling, and comprehensive case management in the care of HIV-infected drug treatment clients. This is discussed in further detail in Chapter 6. Patients can benefit from coordination of care by drug treatment and HIV medical staff. The provision of drug treatment in itself enhances individuals' chances of maintaining their health, while it also makes possible treatment of medical problems and assistance with practical difficulties.

CONCLUSION

The stigma surrounding injection drug users has been deepened by the spread of HIV among their ranks. That stigma extends to those who have sexual relationships with injection drug users. Programs to stem the epidemic among this group will not spring from empathy for their woes. Consequently, it has been and continues to be an important task for researchers and drug treatment providers to demonstrate to policy makers and the public that positive steps can and should be taken to arrest the spread of HIV in this risk population. As a group, we hope that this volume will make a contribution to this end.

Chapter 3

Needle Sharing, Needle Cleaning, and Risk Behavior Change among Injection Drug Users

JOSEPH R. GUYDISH
EVE GOLDEN
KAREN HEMBRY

Injection drug use is the primary risk factor reported in 21% of all adult AIDS cases, with an additional 7% reported among gay men who also inject drugs. The proportion of AIDS cases attributed directly to injection drug use is substantially higher for African-Americans (39%) and Hispanics (40%). Well over half of all heterosexually transmitted cases and pediatric cases are among sexual partners and children of injection drug users (Centers for Disease Control, 1990a).

Successful and sustained behavior change among injection drug users is vital in slowing the spread of HIV in the United States. The ideal behavior change for this population is the discontinuation of drug use, usually through participation in drug treatment. As an overall strategy in slowing the spread of HIV, however, drug treatment is limited. Treatment is inadequate to meet demand, and the provision of "treatment on demand" does not appear to be forthcoming. Current drug treatment resources would have to increase 10-fold in order to accommodate the estimated 1.2 million U.S. injection drug abusers (Presidential Commission on the Human Immunodeficiency Virus Epidemic, 1988). Moreover, many drug users do not enter drug treatment, closing this as an avenue for prevention. Fewer than a quarter of injection drug users are in drug treatment, and some express no interest in entering treatment (Guydish, Temoshok, Dilley, & Rinaldi, 1990b; Jackson, Rotkiewicz, Quinones, & Passannante, 1989; Watters, 1987). For those who do enter drug treatment and fail, or relapse to drug use after a period of abstinence, treatment programs offer only time-limited protection from risk behaviors.

Consequently, effective HIV prevention must include innovative strategies using multiple points of entry into injector communities and targeting specific risk behaviors. This chapter is devoted to HIV risk behavior related to needle use practices. Sexual risk behavior, a vector for HIV transmission that has received little attention among injection drug users, is considered in Chapter 4.

This chapter first reviews the social context of injection drug use, the behaviors that place injection drug users at risk for HIV infection, and factors associated with infection rates (seroprevalence) among injection drug users. Next we consider changes in seroprevalence, and changes in needle-sharing and needle-cleaning behavior, for injection drug user populations in New York and San Francisco. This is followed by a discussion of the nature and types of current interventions designed to reduce risk behavior among injection drug users. Finally, we consider public health implications based on the available studies of risk behavior change.

THE SOCIAL CONTEXT OF INJECTION DRUG USE AND RISK BEHAVIOR

Although the injection drug user population is heterogeneous with respect to drug use patterns and lifestyles, the sharing of injection equipment is common. Needle sharing is often a part of the initiation process, in which new drug users learn injection practices in the presence of experienced users (Powell, 1973; Harding & Zinberg, 1977), and nearly all injection drug users report having shared needles at some time (Lange et al., 1988). Once individuals learn to inject themselves, needle sharing may be maintained as a part of drug-using activity because of various social and environmental factors.

Entry into the injection drug culture involves a socialization process in which the habits, rituals, expectations, and means of survival are learned and shared within the group (Hopkins, 1988). Individuals in these groups tend to be marginalized or excluded by the larger society, and are bound together in systems of mutual support, obligation, and interdependence (Feldman & Biernacki, 1988). Pragmatic benefits are derived from sharing such resources as living accommodations, food, drugs, and injection equipment. The sharing of scarce resources also serves social functions by which bonding and group cohesiveness are affirmed and maintained, and sharing may provide a sense of successful cooperation within a hostile environment (Des Jarlais, 1988b). Individuals who violate or refuse to conform to sharing norms may run the risk of being distrusted and ostracized by a friendship network on which they depend for daily survival needs.

Issues related to gender and sex roles may also affect needle sharing. Historically, the injection-drug-using subculture has been predominantly male-oriented, with a male–female ratio of approximately 5:1 (Lex, 1990). Female injectors are more likely than their male counterparts to have sex partners who inject drugs (Nemoto, Brown, Foster, & Chu, 1990b). Within the subculture is a hierarchy of roles based on gender differences. Men often initiate women into injection drug use and often "fix" women partners, a pattern that continues throughout the drug-using career for some women. To the degree that men occupy the dominant role in such relationships, they are more likely to inject themselves first before sharing with their female sexual partners. Because of the male–female ratio within the subculture, men may have a larger sharing network than women. Consequently, women sharing needles only with their sexual partners have little control over the number of persons with whom their male partners may be sharing.

Environmental factors also have an impact on needle sharing. In several states where the possession of injection equipment is a criminal offense, carrying or keeping needles on hand places the user at risk for arrest and incarceration. The availability of needles as a consumer good also influences sharing, such that when needles are scarce, needle sharing among needle users increases (Feldman & Biernacki, 1988). In addition, variations in the type and quality of drugs used (e.g., China White vs. the more gummy Mexican Black Tar heroin) may influence sharing, by differentially affecting the usable life of syringes and needles. It is within this complex context, replete with social, environmental, subcultural, legal, and sex-role considerations, that HIV prevention efforts targeting injection drug users operate.

FACTORS ASSOCIATED WITH HIV INFECTION

This section discusses two general and consistent findings concerning HIV infection among injection drug users. The first is that infection rates are relatively higher in African-American and Hispanic populations. The second is the relationship between cocaine use and HIV infection.

HIV in Minority Communities

Among the heterosexual injector population, the HIV epidemic has had a devastating and disproportionate effect on African-Americans and

Hispanics. Of all adult AIDS cases attributed to injection drug use (including gay men who also inject drugs), 50% have been African-American, 29% Hispanic, and 20% white (Centers for Disease Control, 1990a). The relative risk of HIV infection for both African-American and Hispanic males is 20 times that of white males (Selik, Castro, & Pappaioanou, 1988). The relative risk for African-American females is 18 times, and for Hispanic females is 10 times, that of white females. Although the high and disproportionate percentage of AIDS cases within minority communities has been attributed to a higher incidence of injection drug use, African-American injectors sometimes report less needle sharing than do whites (Guydish, Abramowitz, Woods, Black, & Sorensen, 1990a). The discrepancy of lower reported needle sharing among minority injection drug users, who have higher seroprevalence rates, is a perplexing research question and one that hinders development of more effective interventions.

One explanation may be that the needle-sharing network among minority injection drug users is smaller than that among whites. Once the virus is introduced into a small and insulated sharing network, the question of which partners one shares with becomes more important than that of how many partners one shares with. HIV infection can be expected to penetrate more deeply and to spread more quickly within a small but regular sharing network. A second explanation is that, given the greater pervasiveness of injection drug use in some minority communities, the male–female ratio may be more nearly even. This gender parity would mean that minority injectors have a greater chance of exposure to the virus, through injection drug use and through having sex with injection drug users, which would elevate the risk of infection. A third possibility is self-report bias, and relates to the in-treatment nature of most of the samples used in drug user research. Minority individuals may be more inclined to underreport the extent of needle sharing, because of a suspicion of institutions that they perceive as untrustworthy. Viewed within a sociohistorical context, this suspicion is grounded in the experiences that minority communities have had with medical research and public health systems in the past.

Cocaine and HIV

The use of cocaine in both injected and noninjected forms may increase the risk of HIV infection. Drug users who inject cocaine alone, or who inject cocaine and other drugs, are more likely to be HIV-infected (Amsel, Battjes, & Pickens, 1990; Chaisson et al., 1989; Nemoto, Brown, Battjes, & Siddiqui, 1990a). Cocaine injectors typically inject more frequently than other injectors, are more likely to use shooting galleries, and have more needle-sharing partners (Chaisson et al., 1989;

Snyder, Nemeth-Coslett, Myers, & Young, 1990; Wiebel, Guydan, & Chene, 1990). Cocaine may have a direct immunological impact on either the likelihood of transmission or susceptibility to infection (Weiss, 1989). Finally, cocaine injectors may be less likely to clean their needles with bleach (Margolis, Catanzarite, Biernacki, & Feldman, 1990).

The use of crack (smokable cocaine) is also implicated in increased risk behavior. In separate cohort studies in New York and San Francisco, the use of crack predicted HIV seroconversion and increased use of shooting galleries (Schoenbaum, Hartel, & Friedland, 1990), and was associated with increased frequency of cocaine injection (Wolfe, Vranizan, Gorter, Cohen, & Moss, 1990). Among injectors, crack use is associated with increased number of sexual partners (Wolfe et al., 1990) and with having an injection-drug-using sexual partner (Schoenbaum et al., 1990). Among noninjecting drug users, crack use is associated with a high number of sexual partners, with exchanging sex for drugs, and with having sex under the influence of drugs or alcohol (R. E. Fullilove, Fullilove, Bowser, & Gross, 1990a), as well as with having multiple injection-drug-using sexual partners (Weissman, Sowder, & Young, 1990). Finally, crack use has been implicated in increasing rates of syphilis, which may be a cofactor for HIV infection (Quinn et al., 1990; Rolfs, Goldberg, & Sharrar, 1990).

The increased HIV risk associated with cocaine use, and the demographic and behavioral differences between those who use cocaine and those who do not (Chaisson et al., 1989; Nemoto et al., 1990a; Wolfe et al., 1990), make it necessary to develop prevention programs targeting cocaine users. The development of efficacious cocaine treatment protocols, in addition to methadone treatment programs, is essential to the prevention of HIV infection in this population.

Summary

Two factors are consistently associated with increased infection rates among injection drug users. First, African-American and Hispanic injection drug users have higher rates of HIV infection, even while reporting lower rates of needle sharing in some studies. This finding may be due to different patterns of needle sharing related to social networks, the greater pervasiveness of injection drug use in some minority communities, or more frequent underreporting of risk behavior by minority drug users. Second is the use of cocaine. Among injectors, the use of cocaine, either by injection or smoking, is associated with higher rates of HIV infection and more frequent risk behavior (both needle use behavior and sexual behavior). Among drug users who do not inject, the use of smokable cocaine (crack) is associated with high-risk sexual behavior.

CHANGES IN SEROPREVALENCE: NEW YORK AND SAN FRANCISCO

The course of the HIV epidemic among injection drug users can be estimated from changes observed in seroprevalence rates over time, as well as changes in annual seroconversion rates (the proportion of cases at risk who become infected each year). In this section, studies of HIV seroprevalence and seroconversion are reviewed for two comparison cities, New York and San Francisco. These two urban areas represent AIDS epicenters with among the highest annual rates of AIDS cases (57 per 100,000 and 109 per 100,000, respectively), and together account for over 25% of all AIDS cases reported in the United States at the end of 1990 (Centers for Disease Control, 1990a). Reviewing HIV-related findings in these two cities illustrates two different patterns of epidemic spread. HIV infection reached saturation proportions among injection drug users in New York from 1978 to 1984, while remaining relatively low among injection drug users in San Francisco through 1990.

New York City

Des Jarlais et al. (1989a) reviewed trends in HIV infection among injection drug users in Manhattan from 1977 to 1987, based on a series of cross-sectional studies. To estimate seroprevalence in injection drug user samples prior to 1984, the authors tested sera that had been collected and stored in conjunction with medical studies not related to HIV. Seroprevalence estimates for later years were derived from samples of participants in methadone detoxification or treatment programs. The rate of HIV infection in these samples increased rapidly from 9% in 1978 to approximately 60% in 1984, and remained stable at this level through 1987. The authors suggest that there was a slow period of growth from the introduction of HIV into the injector community in the mid-1970s until 1978, followed by a phase of rapid spread from 1978 to 1984; a stable phase was then reached in about 1984. Seroconversion rates (annual rate of new infections) also stabilized at an estimated 7% per year. Des Jarlais et al. attribute the stabilization of HIV infection to the interplay among the rate of new infections, HIV saturation in the drug-using community, the loss of infected users and entrance of new uninfected users into the population, and risk behavior change among injection drug users.

San Francisco

Changes in HIV seroprevalence among injection drug users in San Francisco have not been summarized as clearly as those in New York

City, but can be reconstructed from a series of studies. Watters and Cheng (1987) tested in-treatment and out-of-treatment injection drug users in 1985 and 1986. Seroprevalence was 9% for the total sample, but was higher for the out-of-treatment sample (16%) than for the in-treatment sample (7%). The authors noted that this difference was probably due to a sampling artifact, since the out-of-treatment sample included a higher proportion of gay injection drug users.

Chaisson, Moss, Onishi, Osmond, and Carlson (1987a) investigated the prevalence of HIV among San Francisco injection drug users from 1985 to 1987, in several cross-sectional samples recruited from heroin detoxification or methadone maintenance clinics. The investigators reported a 10% seropositivity rate for the sample drawn in 1985, and noted that participants who shared needles regularly were five times more likely to be seropositive. African-American and Hispanic injectors were more likely to be seropositive after sharing behavior was adjusted for, even though whites reported regular sharing with more persons. In a sample recruited in 1986 and 1987, seropositivity rates were 12% overall, 26% for African-Americans, and 10% for Hispanics (Chaisson et al., 1989). Daily cocaine injectors were six times more likely than those who did not inject cocaine to be seropositive. In a separate publication, the same group reported a 15% seroprevalence rate for those tested in 1987 (Chaisson, Osmond, Moss, Feldman, & Biernacki, 1987b).

Moss et al. (1989) evaluated seroprevalence rates for a cohort tested repeatedly at drug detoxification programs in San Francisco, and compared rates of seroconversion in 1985 and 1987. Of 380 injection drug users who were present at more than one data collection point, 11 seroconverted between 1985 and mid-1987 (421 person-years), giving a seroconversion rate of 2.6% per person-year (ppyr). Seroconversion rates were higher for African-Americans (5.7% ppyr) and Hispanics (3.6% ppyr) than for whites (1.8% ppyr). Comparing seroconversion rates over time, the authors reported a 7% ppyr rate in 1985, decreasing to 2.6% ppyr in 1987.

Summary

The series of studies reported by Des Jarlais et al. (1989a) suggest that HIV entered the New York City injection-drug-using community in the mid-1970s, spread slowly for the first few years, spread rapidly from 1978 to 1984, and then stabilized at an approximate 60% seroprevalence and 7% annual seroconversion rate. Seroprevalence data for San Francisco are relatively more recent, beginning in 1985. In the series of cross-sectional studies, HIV seroprevalence increased from about 10% in 1985 to 15% in 1987, and apparently stabilized at that level (Chaisson et al., 1987a, 1987b, 1989). Seroconversion rates, which reflect how rapidly the virus spreads in a community, decreased over time in both New York and San Francisco (Des Jarlais et al., 1989a; Moss et al., 1989).

CHANGES IN RISK BEHAVIOR: NEW YORK AND SAN FRANCISCO

In order to evaluate the relationship between changes in seroprevalence and changes in risk behavior, this section reviews studies of risk behavior change among injection drug users in the two comparison cities. Studies reviewed in this section are summarized in Table 3.1.

New York City

Des Jarlais, Friedman, and Hopkins (1985a) documented increased demand for sterile injection equipment in two ethnographic studies. In 1983, injection drug users participating in a study using an in-depth interview protocol (n = 18) reported increased demand on the street for new injection equipment. In a 1985 sample of needle sellers (n = 22), 82% reported recent increases in sales of new needles, and about half reported misrepresenting and selling used needles as new. The authors inferred "a sustained increase in the use of new needles among drug users in New York City" (p. 758).

New York City street research workers discovered, in 1985, two new marketing practices with respect to clean needles (Des Jarlais & Hopkins, 1985). One change was described as a "two-for-one" sale, in which needle sellers included an additional needle with the sale of one complete needle and syringe outfit. A second change was the practice of including a "free" needle and syringe with the sale of a bag of heroin. These early ethnographic observations suggest increased demand for sterile injection equipment on the street.

To evaluate risk behavior change directly, researchers interviewed 59 clients in a New York methadone maintenance program in 1984 (Friedman et al., 1987). These participants had been in methadone maintenance treatment for an average of over 7 years, and most (91%) had injected within the past 2 years. For this latter subgroup the average number of injections per month was 33, with heroin and cocaine as the most frequently injected drugs. Of the entire sample, 54% reported changes in needle use behavior to decrease AIDS risk; 31% reported either cleaning needles or increased use of clean needles, and 29% reported decreased needle sharing.

TABLE 3.1. Studies of Behavior Change among Injection Drug Users (IDUs): New York and San Francisco

Study	City	Design	Sample	*n*	Outcome
Des Jarlais, Friedman, and Hopkins (1985)	NY	Ethnographic	Out-of-treatment IDUs Needle sellers	18 22	Self-reported increased demand for new needles Increased sale of new needles
Des Jarlais and Hopkins (1985)	NY	Ethnographic	Needle sellers Drug dealers	[a] [a]	Needle sellers including an extra needle with syringe Drug sellers including a needle with a bag of heroin
Selwyn, Feiner, Cox, Lipshutz, and Cohen (1987)	NY	Cross-section	Methadone detox and maintenance clients	261	63% stopping or decreasing injection due to AIDS
Friedman et al. (1987)	NY	Ethnographic	Methadone maintenance clients	59	54% reported changes in needle use behavior due to AIDS; 31% reported needle cleaning; 29% reported decreased needle sharing
Watters (1987)	SF	Longitudinal	In- and out-of-treatment IDUs	108	59% reported decreased needle sharing; 76% reported using bleach to clean needles; 73% reported change in bleach use over 6-month period
Chaisson, Osmond, Moss, Feldman, and Carlson (1987b)	SF	Cross-section	Two samples of in-treatment IDUs (1985 and 1987)	152 172	41% increase in bleach use for needle cleaning 40% decrease in reports of never using bleach No change in reported needle sharing
Watters (1988)	SF	Ethnographic	IDUs recruited through chain referral	27	Decreased number of needle-sharing partners
Sorenson, Guydish, Costantini, and Batki (1989f)	SF	Longitudinal	Sample of all clients entering drug treatment 1986–1988	303	27% decrease in reported needle sharing; decrease in proportion reporting sharing with two or more partners
Gibson, Wermuth, Lovelle-Drache, Ham, and Sorensen (1989b)	SF	Clinical trial of treatment modality	In-treatment IDUs Non-IDU sex partners	88 45	IDUs who received counseling reported more needle cleaning than did those who received only brochures at 10-day follow-up, but not at 90-day follow-up
Guydish, Abramowitz, Woods, Black, and Sorensen (1990a)	SF	Longitudinal	All admissions to two IDU treatment programs over 2-year period	7,660	22% decrease in reported needle sharing; whites more likely to report needle sharing than African-Americans; cocaine-using IDUs shared more than non-cocaine-using IDUs
Guydish, Temoshok, Dilley, and Rinaldi (1990b)	SF	Program evaluation	Consecutive referrals to HIV-affected drug users; majority white gay men	86	27% reported cleaning needles, and 17% reported stopping or decreasing needle sharing

[a] No sample size reported.

In a study to determine AIDS risk awareness and related behavior change, researchers interviewed 261 injection drug users in 1985 (Selwyn, Feiner, Cox, Lipshutz, & Cohen, 1987). Participants were drawn from a methadone maintenance program and the narcotic detoxification unit of a detention facility. Participants were aware of AIDS risk, were concerned about their own potential infection, and demonstrated good basic AIDS knowledge. Among those at risk after learning about AIDS, 63% reported stopping injection drug use or discontinuing needle-sharing practices due to the risk of AIDS. Primary reasons reported for continued needle sharing were the inaccessibility of sterile injection equipment, and sharing only with close friends or relatives.

San Francisco

In a 1987 ethnographic study, Watters (1988) interviewed 27 injection drug users in San Francisco recruited through a chain referral technique. About half were African-American men; the mean age was 36; and heroin and speed were the most frequent drugs of abuse. Nearly all respondents reported sharing with fewer partners because of the AIDS epidemic, prompting the investigator to suggest that needle-sharing circles in this population may be growing smaller.

Sorensen, Guydish, Costantini, and Batki (1989f) evaluated self-reported needle sharing for injection drug users entering a methadone detoxification clinic from 1986 to 1988. All patients entering treatment reported number of needle-sharing occasions and number of sharing partners in the month preceding treatment. The investigators compared data for all admissions in June of each of the three years ($n = 303$). The proportion reporting any needle sharing decreased from 55% in 1986 to 28% in 1988 ($p < .0001$). The proportion sharing with two or more partners in the month prior to treatment decreased much less, from 18% to 13%.

In a longitudinal study of needle-sharing behavior, all injector clients entering two San Francisco drug detoxification programs over a period of 2 years were asked about needle sharing in the 30 days preceding treatment (Guydish et al., 1990a). The data were partitioned into consecutive 6-month periods to allow comparisons of self-reported needle sharing over time. For both clinics combined ($n = 7{,}660$), the proportion of cases reporting any needle sharing in the past month decreased from 50% in 1986 to 28% in 1988. To control for confounding related to readmission of some cases, logistic analyses predicting needle sharing were completed, using only the first admission for each individual ($n = 5{,}610$). Results indicated that whites were more likely to report needle sharing than were African-Americans, and that injectors who also used cocaine were more likely to share than were those who did not use cocaine.

In the context of a program evaluation, substance-abusing clients were asked about their behavior change in response to the AIDS epidemic (Guydish et al., 1990b). Participants were 86 consecutive referrals to a hospital-based program serving HIV-affected patients who also had a drug problem. About half reported a history of injection drug use, and most were gay white men. Of the total sample, 27% reported cleaning needles in response to the epidemic, while 17% reported having stopped or decreased needle-sharing practices.

In 1986, the MidCity Consortium to Combat AIDS and the Youth Environment Services began promoting the use of household bleach for cleaning needles between injections (Newmeyer, 1988). Bleach in a 10:1 dilution with water had been shown to be effective in reducing virus activity (Resnick, Veren, Salahuddin, Tondreau, & Markham, 1986). In this program, community health outreach workers instructed injection drug users on the street in the proper use of bleach to disinfect needles, and regularly distributed a bleach solution in 1-ounce plastic bottles.

In a preliminary evaluation of the bleach outreach strategy, injection drug users drawn from both in-treatment and out-of-treatment sources were interviewed (Watters, 1987). In baseline interviews conducted in 1986, 90% of participants reported sharing needles and other injection equipment; 20% regularly disinfected needles; and only 3% reported cleaning needles with bleach. Six months after bleach outreach activities were initiated, the outreach workers interviewed 108 injection drug users regarding needle sharing and cleaning. Most respondents (59%) reported sharing less than they had a year earlier, and 76% now reported using bleach to clean needles. The authors suggested that the self-reported increase in bleach use (from 3% to 76%) was associated with the educational activities and bleach distribution conducted by the community health outreach workers.

Chaisson et al. (1987b) recruited samples of injection drug users in 1985 (n = 152) and 1987 (n = 172), and also found increases in needle cleaning with bleach. The proportion reporting any needle sharing (71%) did not change over time. The proportion who usually or always cleaned needles with bleach increased from 6% in 1985 to 47% in 1987, whereas the proportion reporting cleaning needles with alcohol remained stable at 23%. These investigators also attributed the observed changes in bleach use to the efforts of the bleach outreach program.

An intervention study found less promising results regarding needle cleaning. Injection drug users (n = 88) were recruited from a heroin detoxification program, and were randomly assigned either to a brief

HIV risk reduction counseling session or to a control condition where they received only informational brochures (Gibson, Wermuth, Lovelle-Drache, Ham, & Sorensen, 1989b; see also Chapter 8). The counseling intervention was designed to address dimensions of the health belief model, such as perceived threat and response efficacy, self-efficacy, and communication skills regarding risk behavior. Over 70% of the sample were followed up at 10 and 90 days after intervention. Measures included self-reported needle sharing, in addition to questions assessing several health belief dimensions. At the 10-day postintervention interview, injection drug users in the counseling condition more frequently reported needle sterilization than injection drug users in the brochure condition. Although changes concerning response efficacy for sexual risk reduction were maintained at the 90-day follow-up, changes for reported needle sterilization were not.

Relapse to Risky Behavior

Although many studies reviewed have demonstrated the modification of old behaviors (e.g., needle sharing) and the initiation of new behaviors (e.g., needle cleaning with bleach), no published work to date addresses the problem of maintaining HIV-related behavior change among injection drug users. In some urban gay communities, where dramatic changes in HIV-related risk behavior have been reported, recent data point up the danger of relapse to risky behavior. In one cohort of gay men followed from 1984 to 1988, 12% of participants relapsed to unsafe sexual practices following initial behavior change (Ekstrand & Coates, 1990). Concerning needle cleaning and needle sharing among injection drug users, research is necessary to determine rates and predictors of relapse. Intervention strategies may be enhanced through the inclusion of relapse prevention components.

Summary

Ethnographic studies in New York City conducted with injection drug users and street needle vendors indicated AIDS awareness, concern about infection, and accommodations to these concerns by the illicit drug market as early as 1983 (Des Jarlais et al., 1985a; Des Jarlais & Hopkins, 1985). In two studies surveying injection drug users recruited through drug treatment programs, 50–60% of participants reported some attempts at risk reduction, most often decreased needle sharing or increased needle cleaning (Friedman et al. 1987; Selwyn et al., 1987).

In a San Francisco ethnographic study (Watters, 1988), and in one study evaluating an AIDS service program (Guydish et al., 1990b), substance abusers reported decreased risk behavior related to needle sharing. Two studies evaluating changes in needle-sharing behavior for injection drug users entering drug detoxification reported decreases in needle sharing, from about 50% in 1986 to 30% in 1988 (Sorensen et al., 1989f; Guydish et al., 1990a). Two studies evaluating needle-cleaning behavior both before and after the implementation of a street-based bleach education campaign reported dramatic increases in needle cleaning with bleach from 1985 to 1987 (Chaisson et al., 1987b; Watters, 1987). Interestingly, the publication by Chaisson and colleagues reported no change in needle sharing during the study period. One study evaluating behavior change following a brief counseling intervention showed increased needle cleaning at 10 days after intervention, but this finding was not maintained at the 90-day follow-up (Gibson et al., 1989b). Finally, although numerous studies have reported changes in HIV-related risk behavior among injection drug users, few have investigated the stability of these changes or the likelihood of relapse to unsafe needle use practices.

INTERVENTIONS WITH INJECTION DRUG USERS

Discontinuing drug use through participation in drug abuse treatment is the single best HIV prevention strategy, as it confers significant individual benefit on injection drug users, as well as significant public health benefit. The role of drug treatment, particularly for those already infected with HIV, is discussed in Chapter 6. In addition to drug abuse treatment, however, the armamentarium of HIV prevention strategies targeting injection drug users now includes clinic-based interventions (Sorensen et al., 1989f; Gibson et al., 1989b), street outreach projects (Newmeyer, 1988), community-based information and awareness campaigns (Sorensen, Heitzmann, & Guydish, 1990), and needle exchange programs (Stimson, Alldritt, Dolan, & Donoghoe, 1988).

Clinic-based interventions are HIV prevention programs conducted within drug abuse treatment settings. Because drug users know and use drug treatment programs, such programs are an important means of delivering prevention messages. Interventions conducted within substance abuse treatment settings may reach beyond the clients themselves, providing prevention information to family members, friends, and other injection drug users not in treatment (Bixler, Palacios-Jimenez, & Springer, 1987). Examples of clinic-based interventions are described in Chapter 7 (a psychoeducational group format), Chapter 8 (an individual counseling format), and Chapter 9 (clinic-based outreach to injection drug users and sexual partners).

Street outreach programs are designed to deliver prevention messages to injection drug users who may not have regular contact with drug treatment programs or other public health agencies. Outreach workers visit neighborhoods having large injector populations and develop trust with users in the local community through regular face-to-face contact. Workers provide HIV prevention information, referrals to drug treatment or other health and social services, and (in some programs) bleach for needle cleaning. The National Institute on Drug Abuse, through the National AIDS Demonstration Research (NADR) Project, currently supports over 60 outreach programs nationwide, targeting injection drug users and their sexual partners (Nova Research Company, 1989).

Community-based information and awareness campaigns use mass media approaches, targeting a broad audience, to deliver prevention messages. One example is the creation of "Bleachman," an 8-foot tall superhero dressed in a Superman-like costume, with a white bleach bottle for a head. Bleachman, whose mission is to teach people about proper needle cleaning, visits events and fund raisers in the community, and appears on posters, billboards, and television (San Francisco AIDS Foundation, 1988).

Needle exchange programs, in which injection drug users trade used needles for new ones, were instituted in Amsterdam in 1984 and thereafter in several European countries. Beginning in 1988, U.S. needle exchange programs have been initiated in Tacoma and Seattle, Washington; Portland, Oregon; San Francisco; New York City; Boulder, Colorado; and Honolulu, Hawaii (Purchase, Hagan, Des Jarlais, & Reid, 1989; Bolland & Hunter, 1990; Clark et al., 1989; Raymond, 1988a; Schouten et al., 1990). The implementation of exchange programs in the United States has the potential to slow the spread of HIV among injection drug users, their sexual partners, and their children. It is a controversial strategy, however, in that it contradicts traditional wisdom concerning drug treatment and removes at least one barrier to drug use.

PUBLIC HEALTH IMPLICATIONS AND FUTURE DIRECTIONS

Whether the changes observed in the course of the HIV epidemic among injection drug users are related to public health and prevention strategies is unknown, partly because of methodological problems (discussed in Chapter 10), which limit the ability to draw causal inferences. That changes in behavior and seroprevalence are associated with prevention strategies can be asserted, however, based on the consistency of findings and the relationship in time between the introduction of prevention strategies and the changes observed.

Studies in both New York and San Francisco consistently report stabilization of HIV seroprevalence in drug user communities, and they report leveling or decreasing annual seroconversion rates in these communities. Risk behavior change data are also consistent, with substantial changes in needle sharing or needle cleaning reported in nearly every study reviewed. A relationship in time is observable as the result of different infection patterns for New York and San Francisco. HIV entered the New York drug user community sometime in the 1970s (Des Jarlais et al., 1989a), but apparently entered the San Francisco injection-drug-using community a few years later (Watters, 1989). By 1984, when prevention strategies were in operation in both cities, a near-saturation level of infection had already been reached in New York. In San Francisco, however, seroprevalence levels in 1984 were about 10%, and could be affected by prevention strategies. The course of the epidemic among injection drug users in these cities after aggressive prevention interventions began has been similar. Seroprevalence rates appear to have stabilized, although at radically different levels. It appears at this time that the explosive spread of HIV experienced by the New York injection drug user community has been slowed significantly within the San Francisco drug-using community.

Slowing the spread of HIV, although good news, is different from halting the spread. Because the virus is transmitted most effectively from person to person through the injection route, even substantially decreased needle sharing continues to carry significant infection risk and to promote epidemic spread. In San Francisco, for example, an annual seroconversion rate of 2.6% among injection drug users translates into about 300 new cases of HIV infection per year. The implementation of multiple and innovative HIV prevention strategies targeting drug users continues to be a vital public health need. Based on this review, three issues in particular should be used to inform the development of further interventions: (1) the relationship between HIV and cocaine; (2) issues related to HIV in minority communities; and (3) relapse to risky behavior.

Chapter 4

Unsafe Sex and Behavior Change

KYUNG-HEE CHOI
LAURIE A. WERMUTH

Sexual contact has become an increasing cause of HIV infection among heterosexuals. In 1984, only 59 adult heterosexual transmission cases were reported to the Centers for Disease Control (CDC). The annual incidence of heterosexual transmission, however, rose steadily, reaching 1,954 new cases in 1989. As of December 31, 1990, a total of 4,440 cases were attributed to heterosexual contact, comprising 5% of all the adult AIDS cases in the United States (CDC, 1984, 1991).

Injection drug users have played a major role in spreading HIV among heterosexuals. Of the 8,440 heterosexual transmission cases reported through 1990, 53% (4,470 cases) were people who had sexual contact with injection drug users. In addition, indirect HIV transmission by injection drug users has occurred among infants. By the end of 1990, there were 2,786 pediatric AIDS cases. Of these, 21% (487 cases) were infants whose mothers were sexual partners of drug injectors.

Despite injection drug users' direct and indirect role in heterosexual transmission of HIV, only recently has much attention been paid to the issues of sexual behaviors in the injection-drug-using population. This chapter discusses AIDS risk sexual behaviors and obstacles to behavioral changes among injection drug users and their sexual partners. The first section describes patterns of heterosexual HIV transmission by injection drug users. Next come descriptions of AIDS risk sexual practices, AIDS risk perception, changes in sexual behaviors, and difficulties associated with risk reduction. The chapter ends with a discussion of public health implications and future research.

THE PATTERN OF HETEROSEXUAL HIV TRANSMISSION BY INJECTION DRUG USERS

The distribution of AIDS cases among injection drug users shows that women and African-Americans are overrepresented. In addition, seroprevalence studies reveal the highest infectivity among injection drug users as compared to other risk groups, and male-to-female sexual exposure to HIV is more efficient in spreading the disease than female-to-male exposure.

The Distribution of AIDS

The AIDS distribution in the U.S. adult population shows that AIDS cases among men outnumber AIDS cases among women by a ratio of 10:1 (CDC, 1990a). By race, a majority of AIDS cases are whites (56.7%). African-Americans (26.9%) are the next most affected by the epidemic, and Hispanics comprise 15.4% of all AIDS cases.

By comparison, an overwhelming majority of women (71.6%) constitute AIDS cases attributed to heterosexual contact with injection drug users, as shown in Table 4.1. The male–female ratio of the number of the AIDS cases among injection drug users is 1:2.5. This ratio seems to indicate that infected male injection drug users are sexually transmitting HIV to their female partners.

The racial distribution shows a predominance of African-Americans in heterosexually transmitted AIDS cases among injection drug users. More than half (56.7%) of all injector-related heterosexual AIDS cases

TABLE 4.1. AIDS Cases Attributed to Heterosexual Contact with Injection Drug Users (IDUs) by Gender and Race, as of December 1989

	Men		Women		Total	
	%	(*n*)	%	(*n*)	%	(*n*)
All	28.4	(232)	71.6	(2,055)	100.0	(2,871)
White	28.4	(232)	19.6	(402)	22.1	(634)
Black	56.7	(463)	48.2	(991)	50.6	(1,454)
Hispanic	14.6	(119)	31.3	(643)	26.5	(762)
Other	0.3	(2)	0.9	(19)	0.8	(21)
Total	100.0	(816)	100.0	(2,055)	100.0	(2,871)

Note. From *HIV/AIDS Surveillance Report* by the Centers for Disease Control, 1990, January, Atlanta: Author.

are African-Americans. Hispanics, on the other hand, represent 26.5% of the cases, and whites constitute 22.1%. This distribution of heterosexual cases may reflect the finding that African-Americans and Hispanics inject drugs more frequently than whites (CDC, 1989). Some have speculated that they also may share needles more (Peterson & Marin, 1988; however, some studies reviewed in Chapter 2 have found the opposite), and in turn may be more likely to get infected with HIV. For example, the HIV antibody testing of 291 injection drug users recruited in San Francisco showed that African-Americans and Hispanics were almost three times more likely to be HIV-positive than whites (Chaisson, Moss, Onishi, Osmond, & Carlson, 1987a). In addition, Peterson and Bakeman (1989) speculated that low access to sterile drug equipment and the poor health status of minority groups may contribute to higher proportions of AIDS cases among African-Americans and Hispanics.

When the gender- and race-specific proportion of heterosexual AIDS cases is considered, an interesting pattern emerges. The ratios of men to women obtained from Table 4.1 are similar for whites (1:2.1) and for African-Americans (1.7:1). Among Hispanics, however, the ratio is much higher (1:5.4). Hispanic women are 5.4 times more likely to be heterosexual AIDS cases than Hispanic men. This ethnic difference may lie in cultural values influencing sexual behavior. One possible explanation may be that Hispanic cultures discourage female initiation of protective sexual practices (such as condom use) to a greater extent than other cultural groups in the United States (Poma, 1987).

HIV Prevalence

Since clinical manifestation of AIDS may take an average of 8 to 10 years (Medley, Anderson, Cox, & Billard, 1987; Lui, Darrow, & Rutherford, 1988), AIDS surveillance data may not provide an accurate picture of current HIV transmission. Although the precise prevalence of HIV-infected heterosexuals is not known, estimates of seroprevalence rates can give us insights into current transmission patterns. For example, Table 4.2 reveals marked variations of seroprevalence rates by risk groups. HIV infectivity remains highest among injection drug users, followed by sexual partners of HIV-infected persons. Newborn infants in the general population and heterosexuals without known risk factors experience low prevalence of HIV transmission.

INJECTION DRUG USERS

HIV seroprevalence among injection drug users differs by geographic location. New York City, northern New Jersey, and Puerto Rico have

TABLE 4.2 Selected Seroprevalence in the Heterosexual Population

Population	Area	Sample	Year	Percent positive
Injection drug users				
Injection drug users entering treatment (Des Jarlais et al., 1989)	New York City	559	1984–87	57
Injection drug users not in treatment (Williams, 1990)	Houston, Texas	921	NA	8
Injection drug users in methadone maintenance (San Francisco Department of Public Health, 1990)	San Francisco	966	1989–90	9
Heterosexual partners of HIV-infected persons				
Sexual partners of AIDS patients (CDC, 1989)	New York City	114	1982–88	45
Sexual parters of IDUs in detoxification (Moore, Padian,Vranizan, Brodie, & Moss, 1990)	California	29	1988–89	34
Female sexual partners of HIV-positive men (Padian et al.,1987)	California	97	1987	23
Newborn infants				
Newborns given metabolic screening (Novick et al., 1989)	New York City	125,120	1987–88	1.25 all 0.13 for white 1.82 for black 1.31 for Hispanic
Infants providing umbilical-cord blood samples (Landesman, Minkoff, Holman, McCalla, & Sijin, 1987)	New York City	602	1986–87	2.00
Heterosexuals without known risk factors				
Women seeking maternity services (Weisenfus, Back, & O'Hara, 1988)	New York City	2,162	1987	1.4
Enlisted U.S. Army soldiers (Kelly et al., 1990)	All states	648,032	1985–89	0.25 all 0.26 for men 0.11 for women 0.13 for white 0.51 for black 0.40 for Hispanic
Civilian female applicants for military service (Gayle, Selik, & Chu, 1990)	All states	358,584	1985–89	0.06 all 0.02 for white 0.15 for black 0.08 for Hispanic

reported injection drug user infection rates as high as 60% (Turner, Miller, & Moses, 1989). In particular, among those entering drug treatment centers in Manhattan (New York City) between 1984 and 1987, 57% were HIV-positive (Des Jarlais et al., 1989a). Infection rates in other parts of the country, such as Houston, Texas (8%) and San Francisco, California (9%), are much lower (Williams, 1990; San Francisco Department of Public Health AIDS Office, 1990).

HETEROSEXUAL PARTNERS OF PERSONS AT RISK

HIV prevalence among heterosexual partners of HIV-infected persons varies by their level of AIDS risk. Among heterosexual partners of AIDS patients, seroprevalence was 45% (CDC, 1989). The rate of HIV infection among female partners of injection drug users was 34% (Moore, Padian, Vranizan, Brodie, & Moss, 1990). A study by Padian et al. (1987) found a relatively low rate of infection; of 97 women who were sexual partners of HIV-infected men, 23% were HIV-positive.

NEWBORN INFANTS

A seroprevalence study of 602 umbilical-cord blood samples from infants delivered at one inner-city municipal hospital in New York between December 1986 and January 1987 revealed a seroprevalence of 2% (12 of 602). Of those tested, 58% of the mothers acknowledged intravenous drug use or sexual contact with people at risk for AIDS (Landesman, Minkoff, Holman, McCalla, & Sijin, 1987; Minkoff et al., 1988). A survey of maternal HIV antibodies conducted in New York State reported a HIV seroprevalence rate of 1.25% statewide. An examination of seroprevalence by ethnicity showed that 0.13% were whites, 1.82% were African-Americans, and 1.31% were Hispanics (Novick et al., 1989).

HETEROSEXUALS WITHOUT KNOWN AIDS RISK

Between 1985 and 1989, the U.S. Army screened most active-duty soldiers for the HIV antibody. Of 648,032 enlisted personnel who received test results, 1,588 (0.25%) were infected with HIV (Kelley et al., 1990). There were 1,516 HIV-positive men and 72 HIV-positive women. Seroprevalence rates were higher among those aged 25–29 (0.31%) and aged 30–34 (0.34%) than among those aged 20–24 (0.18%) and those older than 34 (0.22%). African-Americans (0.51%) and Hispanics (0.40%) had higher infection rates than whites (0.13%).

During the same period, a total of 358,584 female applicants for military service received HIV antibody testing (Gayle, Selik, & Chu, 1990). Those applicants showed a lower infection rate (0.06%) compared to enlisted personnel in the U.S. Army. Seroprevalence was again higher for African-Americans (0.15%) and Hispanics (0.08%) than for whites (0.02%).

Efficacy of Heterosexual Transmission

May and Anderson (1987) postulated that the future course of the heterosexual epidemic would depend on three major parameters: (1) the number of sexual contacts between infected men and susceptible women and between infected women and susceptible men; (2) rates of acquiring new partners of the other sex by women and men; and (3) the time from HIV infection to manifestation of AIDS symptoms. They showed that should the rate of secondary transmission determined by these three parameters exceed 1, heterosexual infection of HIV would grow exponentially.

A lack of reliable data makes it difficult to judge whether we will witness the exponential growth of heterosexual transmission in the future. A few studies available, in the meantime, indicate that heterosexual transmission occurs more frequently among those who inject drugs than among those who do not. As Table 4.3 shows, Padian and colleagues (1987) recruited 97 women who were sexual partners of 93 men infected with HIV in California. In their sample, 23% tested HIV-positive. By risk groups, female partners of bisexuals (22%), hemophiliacs (21%), and men infected from contaminated transfusions (25%) reported similar infection rates. By contrast, seropositivity for female partners of injection drug users was almost twice as high (42%). Another study was able to locate 19 women and 10 men who were sexual partners of 68 seropositive injection drug users (Moore et al., 1990). In that study, 34% were infected with HIV.

Studies of the efficiency of heterosexual transmission reveal that female partners of seropositive men have higher infection rates than male partners of seropositive women. Padian, Shiboski, and Jewell (1990) interviewed 41 male sexual partners of HIV-infected women and 219 female sexual partners of HIV-infected men in 1985–1989. The infection rate for the former group was 2.4%, whereas 20% of the latter group were HIV-positive. The estimated odds ratio showed that the male-to-female transmission was 12 times higher than the female-to-male transmission. Evidence available from Italy also suggests this trend. Among 106 steady female sexual partners of HIV-positive men followed from 1986 to 1989, 5.7% were infected with the virus. In the

TABLE 4.3 The Efficiency of Heterosexual Transmisson

Study	Sample	Transmission rate (%)
Padian (1987)	97 female sexual partners of 93 HIV+ men	23
Padian (1989)	10 HIV+ IDUs	20
Moore (1990)	29 sexual partners of IDUs in detoxification	34
Padian, Shiboski, & Jewell (1990)	41 male sexual partners of 38 HIV+ women	2.4 2.4
Alberto (1990)	158 women with steady partners of HIV+ men	3.8
Tacconi et. al. (1990)	106 HIV+ men with steady female partners 36 HIV+ women with steady male partners	5.7 0.0

same period, none of the steady male partners of 36 HIV-positive women had become seropositive (Tacconi et al., 1990).

AIDS RISK SEXUAL BEHAVIORS AMONG INJECTION DRUG USERS AND SEXUAL PARTNERS

A dearth of comparable data on sexual behavior of drug users and nonusers makes AIDS risk assessment difficult. To date, there are two national surveys of sexual behavior in the adult population of the United States: the 1988 General Social Survey conducted by the National Opinion Research Center (n = 1,481) and the 1987 *Los Angeles Times Survey* (n = 2,095) (Turner et al., 1989). For the drug injection population, no one has conducted such large-scale studies. Information on injection drug users' sexual behavior comes primarily from surveys of drug users in drug rehabilitation clinics and evaluation studies of AIDS prevention programs. Reviews of current data suggest that injection drug users are at a higher risk of sexual exposure to HIV than the general public. The sexual partners of injection drug users face considerable risk of exposure and HIV infection.

Sexual Practices

The National Opinion Research Center conducted face-to-face interviews with a probability sample of 1,481 adults residing in U.S. households in 1988 (Michael, Laumann, Gagnon, & Smith, 1988). According to the survey, 21.5% of the respondents had had no sex partner in the past 12 months, 59.6% had had one, and 12.8% had had two or more. Two other studies yielded similar estimates. A national survey of 2,095 adults conducted by the Los Angeles Times in 1987 found 15% without sex partners 12 months prior to the interview, 70% with one partner, and 15% with two or more partners (Turner et al., 1989). Among 1,842 women aged 15–44 randomly selected in New York City, 28.8% reported having had no partner within the past year, while 59.8% indicated having had one steady partner, and 11.4% said two or more (Fordyce, Balanon, & Stoneburner, 1990).

By comparison, it seems that injection drug users are at higher risk for AIDS than the general population. Table 4.4 shows that the proportion of injection drug users with multiple partners ranges from 31% to as high as 83%, depending on samples. Magura, Shapiro, Siddiqi, and Lipton (1990), for example, found that 31% of 211 injection drug users enrolled in methadone maintenance programs in New York City had had two or more sexual partners in the past year. Lewis, Watters, and Case (1990) reported even a higher proportion of injection drug users with multiple sexual partners among those either in or out of drug treatment. Their sample of 149 men with stable female partners in San Francisco showed that 83% of the respondents reported having had two or more female sexual partners during the past 5 years. This figure is even higher than that for some samples of homosexuals. For example, the 1989 population-based sample of 300 gay and bisexual men in Los Angeles County showed that 53% had had more than one partner (Yano, Gorman, Kanouse, Berry, & Abrahamse, 1990).

Some drug injectors practice heterosexual anal intercourse and engage in bisexual behavior. Lewis et al. (1990) interviewed 70 white and 79 African-American men in San Francisco who injected drugs and had regular sexual partners. Of their 149 subjects, 38% reported having anal intercourse. Whites (46%) were more likely to perform anal intercourse than African-Americans (30%). In another sample of 336 injection drug users surveyed in San Francisco, 13% were bisexuals (Lewis & Watters, 1990). Of the bisexuals, 12% reported heterosexual anal intercourse, and 33% reported homosexual anal intercourse. Of the heterosexuals, 12% also said that they had had heterosexual anal intercourse.

In addition, a substantial number of injection drug users are engaged in prostitution. Lewis and Watters (1991) analyzed the 1987 targeted sample of 457 whites and African-Americans recruited from treatment and street settings in San Francisco. Their analysis showed that 35% gave sex in exchange for money or drugs. Female respondents (50%) more often reported prostitution than male respondents (26%). African-American respondents (42%) were more likely to be involved in prostitution than were white respondents (28%). By race and gender, African-American women (58%) reported the highest prevalence of

TABLE 4.4. Selected Study Findings of IDUs Sexual Behaivor

Study	Sample	Sexual behavior
D.L. Murphy (1987)	1986 representative sample of 93 attending methadone maintenance clinics in New York City	60% had two or more partners during 1977–1985 66% had sexual contacts with non-IDUs (70% of men; 40% of women)
Lewis, Watters, & Case (1990)	1987 sample of 149 male IDUs with stable partners in San Francisco	63% had two or more partners in last year; 40% had sexual contacts with non-IDUs 73% never used condoms
Jain et al.	1987 convenience sample of 671 attending an AIDS prevention program in Sacramento, CA	Three to six partners on average 1 and 6 months prior to interview 68% never used condoms
Sotheran et al. (1989)	1987–1988 convenience sample of 137 attending methadone maintenance clinics in New York City	43% had two or more partners 44% never used condoms
Magura, Shapiro, Siddiqi, & Lipton (1990)	1987–1988 convenience sample of 211 attending methadone maintenance clinic in New York City	31% had two or more partners 67% had sexual contacts with non-IDUs
Lewis & Watters (1990)	1989 targeted sample of 336 male IDUs in San Francisco	40% had two or more partners 61% never used condoms 21% exchanged sex for drugs and money
Kroliczak (1990)	1990 national sample of 5,280 female sexual partners of IDUs	51% of non-IDUs and 57% of IDUs had two or more partners 61% of both non-IDUs and IDUs never used condoms
Pappas, Gaulard, Winterhalter, & Christen (1990)	1989 convenience sample of 100 female sexual partners of IDUs in San Francisco	33% prostituted for money 72% never used condoms

prostitution. However, it may be that African-American women as a group are more willing to self-report prostitution than their white counterparts.

Despite a high awareness about sexual transmission of AIDS, unprotected sexual practices are still pervasive both in the drug-using and non-drug-using populations. In an analysis of the 1987 Los Angeles Times survey of 2,095 adults, Turner and colleagues (1989) found that a larger number of sexually active men (45% reporting nine or more partners during the past year) and women (65% reporting three or more partners) stated that they had never purchased condoms during the past year.

In the drug-using population, Lewis and Watters (1990) found that a majority (61%) never used condoms in their sexual practices. Three other studies found comparable proportions of condom use among injection drug users. Lewis and colleagues (1990) reported that 73% of 149 injection drug users in San Francisco had never used condoms in the past year, while Jain and colleagues (1989) found that 68% of their sample of 671 injectors in Sacramento, California had never used condoms in the last month. In the sample of 211 injection drug users interviewed by Magura et al. (1990) in New York City, 68% had not used condoms at all during the previous month. By race and gender, Lewis and Watters (1991) found little difference in condom use between whites (66% never using condoms) and African-Americans (69% never using condoms), and also between men (58% never using condoms) and women (61% never using condoms) in their sample of 457 injection drug users interviewed in San Francisco.

Many injection drug users have sexual contacts outside the drug-using group, and therefore can transmit the virus to their noninjecting sexual partners. In particular, men who inject drugs, if infected, can transmit the virus to many women who are their sexual partners. Des Jarlais, Chamberland, Yancovitz, Weinberg, and Friedman (1984) interviewed 50 injection drug users entering the inpatient drug detoxification program in New York City. All of the respondents except one had long-term heterosexual relationships that had lasted almost 6 years on average. A majority of them (78%) had steady relationships with women who did not inject drugs. Similarly, Magura et al.'s (1990) study of 211 injection drug users in methadone maintenance (1990) found that 67% of the sample had sexual contacts with noninjectors.

In D. L. Murphy's (1987) survey of a representative sample of 93 clients in methadone treatment, a similar proportion had heterosexual partners who were not drug injectors (68%). In her sample, men (70%) were more likely to have non-drug-using sex partners than women (40%). Among those who shared no needles, similar proportions of men (68%) and women (68%) reported sexual contacts with noninjectors. Among those who shared needles, noninjector sexual contacts were significantly more frequent for men (78%) than for women (22%).

To assess AIDS risk among female sexual partners of injection drug users, the National Institute on Drug Abuse's National AIDS Demonstration Research (NADR) Project surveyed 5,280 such women (Kroliczak, 1990). This survey found that 3,347 (63%) had injected drugs themselves, and the rest (1,933) had never injected drugs. Among female sexual partners who had no history of drug use, 51% had had more than one partner and 61% never used condoms. Comparable proportions of drug-using women (57% with multiple partners and 61%

not using condoms) reported similar sexual behavior. This survey also found that 42% of injection-drug-using female partners and 30% of noninjecting female partners had traded sex for money or drugs. Over three-quarters of those trading sex for money or drugs reported either never or sometimes using condoms.

Pappas, Gaulard, Winterhalter, and Christen (1990) interviewed 100 female sexual partners of injection drug users in San Francisco between May and September 1989. Their sample demonstrated a high level of knowledge about HIV transmission, but only a few of survey respondents practiced "safer sex." About three out of four never used condoms either with their primary sexual partners or secondary sexual partners. Moreover, 33% of the sample traded sex for money, and 11% identified themselves as prostitutes.

AIDS Risk Perception

Weinstein (1987), Mays and Cochran (1988), and Cochran (1989) all stress the importance of one's perception of AIDS risk in behavior change. Cochran (1989), in particular, has argued that motivation to alter sexual practices depends on the perception of risk, and that accurate perception in turn may change risky behavior.

Many injection drug users and their female sexual partners do not perceive themselves at risk for AIDS. D. R. Gibson (personal communication, 1990) surveyed a sample of 226 injection drug users recruited for an AIDS prevention program in San Francisco. According to his study, only a third of the injection drug users interviewed reported being "considerably" or "extremely" troubled by "thoughts that they might be carrying the AIDS virus." A similar proportion (31%) of those in Magura and colleagues' (1990) sample assessed that they were at risk of contracting AIDS. In a study of women sexual partners of injection drug users (Wermuth, Choi, Ham, Falcone, & Hulley, 1991), respondents were asked, "In your current relationship(s), do you think you are at risk for AIDS?" Thirty-nine percent of the 77 study participants answered "no."

The low level of perception among injection drug users may be attributable to their unstable, risk-taking life circumstances. Mays and Cochran (1988) point out that poor African-American and Hispanic women, in particular, may rate AIDS as low relative to other risks threatening their well-being. Most women living in poverty may be most worried about their immediate survival and basic needs such as food and shelter. Physical abuse and violence may be of top concern for some. For example, in a survey of 50 female drug users, prostitutes, and runaway youths in San Francisco neighborhoods, more than half

(52%) mentioned violence and drug contacts in their lives, but only 9 (18%) mentioned AIDS as a risk (Derby & Lovelle-Drache, 1990).

The lack of knowledge about sexual partners' drug use and HIV seropositivity may also contribute to the low level of perception. Injection drug users infected with HIV may be reluctant to disclose their serostatus to their partners, fearing rejection and abandonment (Peterson & Marin, 1988). In particular, many female sexual partners of injection drug users may not realize that they are at risk for HIV infection. Wermuth's data (Wermuth et al.,1991) showed that 10% of her sample (8 out of the 77 women sexual partners of injectors interviewed) did not know whether their male partners were currently injecting drugs; 13% (10 out of 77) did not know whether their partners had been tested for HIV antibody.

Changes in Sexual Behaviors

Numerous studies have documented dramatic changes in injection behavior among injection drug users, as discussed in Chapter 3. One recent study (Watters et al., 1990) analyzed six cross-sections of injection drug users tested for HIV status in San Francisco between 1986 ($n = 363$) and 1989 ($n = 228$). The percentage of injection drug users who did not share needles increased from 9% in 1986 to 35% in 1989. For the same period, more drastic changes occurred in the use of safe needle hygiene (13% to 73%) and bleach use (3% to 86%).

Although injection drug users have made significant improvements in needle use, an overwhelming majority seem to experience difficulties in sexual behavior. Table 4.5 illustrates the lack of consistent evidence for changes in sexual behavior among injection drug users. Curtis and colleagues (1989), Schilling and colleagues (1989b), and Abdul-Ouader and colleagues (1989), for example, found about half of their samples reporting changes in sexual behavior. Also, Chitwood et al. (1990b) and Saxon and Calsyn (1990) showed their AIDS prevention programs as being effective in risk reduction. By contrast, among those injection drug users interviewed in 1988 ($n = 243$) and in 1990 ($n = 126$) interviewed by Van den Hoek and van Haastrecht (1990) in Amsterdam, The Netherlands, few had modified their behavior in terms of condom use. Thirty-nine percent of men and 32% of women reported some condom use in 1988, whereas in 1990 38% of men and 25% of women reported some condom use. The same was true for casual sexual contacts: 33% of men and 19% of women had casual sexual partners in 1988, whereas 27% of men and 26% of women had casual sexual partners in 1990. Kall and Olin (1990) also observed little change in condom use among injection drug users arrested and detained in Stockholm, Sweden (74% nonusers in 1987 and 70% nonusers in 1988).

TABLE 4.5. Selected Study Findings of Sexual Behavior Change in Injection Drug Users

Study	Sample	Sexual behavior
Schilling et al. (1989b)	248 IDUs in methadone treatment, New York/northern New Jersey	50% changed sexual behavior in past 6 months
Abdul-Ouader et al. (1989)	279 male IDUs in New York City neighborhoods	55% reported making one or more sexual behavioral changes because of AIDS
Jain et al. (1989)	671 IDUs in AIDS prevention program interviewed at baseline and 4- to 6- month follow-up	68% never used condoms at baseline, and 64% never used them at follow-up An average of 3–11 sexual partners at baseline, but 2–6 at follow-up
Chitwood et al. (1990b)	400 IDUs in AIDS prevention program interviewed at baseline and 6-month follow-up, Miami, Florida	55% decreased but 21% increased number of drug-injecting sex partners Increase in condom use from 32% to 51%
Saxon & Calson (1990)	65 IDUs with multiple partners in AIDS prevention program interviewed at baseline and 6-month follow-up, Seattle, Washington	59% became non-promiscuous
Watters et al. (1990)	3,441 IDUs tested for HIV antibody during 1986–1989, San Francisco	3% used condoms in 1986; 15% in 1987; 21% in 1988; 22% in 1989
Kall & Olin (1990)	40 arrested and detained IDUs in Stockholm, Sweden between 1987–1988	74% never used condoms in 1987, and 70% never used them in 1988
Van den Hoek & van Haastrecht (1990)	243 IDUs interviewed in 1988 and 1990, Amsterdam, The Netherlands	39% of men and 32% of women used condoms in 1988, but 38% of men and 25% of women used them in 1990 33% of men and 19% of women had casual sexual contact in 1988, but 27% of men and 26% of women reported the same behavior in 1990

There are many studies contending that injection drug users are more resistant to changing their sexual behavior than to changing their needle-sharing practices (Battjes & Pickens, 1988; Casadonte, Des Jarlais, Friedman, & Rotrosen, 1988; Des Jarlais & Friedman, 1988; Flynn et al., 1988; Friedman et al., 1987; Jain et al., 1989; Mosley, Kramer, Cancelliari, & Ottomenelli, 1988; Primm, Brown, Gibson, & Chum, 1988; Schilling et al., 1989b). In a first study of injection drug users in methadone maintenance, Friedman and associates (1987) showed that only 14% of the subjects modified their sexual behavior, while 54% changed their drug injection behavior. A more recent study (Jain et al., 1989) of injection drug users in the AIDS prevention program in Sacramento, California showed a drastic decrease in needle sharing from 93% at baseline to 66% at the 6-month follow-up. Few, however, reported using condoms. At baseline, 68% never used condoms; at follow-up, 64% still did not use them.

The difficulty in changing sexual behavior is not unique to injection drug users. Even among the San Francisco gay men for whom dramatic behavior changes have been documented, sexual risk taking persists. Many gay men experience relapse from safer sex, despite massive community campaigns against risk-taking sexual behaviors. According to Stall, Ekstrand, Pollack, and Coates (1990a), 19% of those who practiced only safe sex in 1987 reported engaging in unprotected anal intercourse in the following year. Ekstrand and Coates (1990) also found that 12% of the subjects in the San Francisco Men's Health Study practiced unprotected receptive anal intercourse during a period following initial behavior change.

OBSTACLES TO RISK REDUCTION

Despite ongoing AIDS prevention campaigns, injection drug users still confront many difficulties in modifying their sexual behavior. Addiction and negative attitudes toward condoms have hampered their risk reduction efforts. Economic and emotional dependence, and lack of partner communication and cooperation, enhance the danger of AIDS—particularly among women partners of male injection drug users. The imbalance of power within intimate relationships makes it difficult to negotiate behavioral changes without risking the loss of the relationships. In addition, AIDS stigma and denial of risk drive many injection drug users into isolation and reduce the possibility of seeking early treatment.

Substance Use

Substance use during sex has been shown to reduce compliance with safe sex guidelines for AIDS (Buffum, 1988; Mondanaro, 1987; Stall, McKusick, Wiley, Coates, & Ostrow, 1986). Stall and associates (1986) reported in their analysis of gay men in San Francisco that the use of drugs (e.g., marijuana, "poppers") during sex, the number of drugs used during such activity, and the frequency of combining drugs and sex were all positively associated with risky sexual activity.

In a study of young sexually active women, Eversley (personal communication, February 12, 1991) found a high proportion consuming alcohol and drugs during sex. Her data were collected in San Francisco Bay Area Planned Parenthood Clinics (92 whites and 93 African-Americans). The study found that 54% of whites and 46% of African-Americans consumed alcohol during sex; 21% of whites and 18% of African-Americans used drugs during sex. Both whites and African-Americans who combined substance use and sex practiced more unsafe sex with their sexual partners.

No direct effect of substance use during sex has been investigated for injection drug users. Nonetheless, if alcohol and drugs are used to enhance sexual pleasure, they are likely to decrease judgment and pain sensitivity. The consequence would be difficulties in following safer sex instructions and increases in risk for HIV infection. Earlier studies in New York (Marmor et al., 1987) and in San Francisco (Chaisson et al., 1987a) have already established the positive association between injection drug use and HIV seropositivity. A more recent study of 302 injection drug users in Seattle indicated that less frequent drug injection was associated with less risky sexual behavior (Calsyn, Saxon, & Freeman, 1990).

Attitudes toward Condom Use

Several studies (e.g., Arnold, 1972; Darrow, 1974; Finkel & Finkel, 1975) have identified a number of obstacles to condom use among patients at sexually transmitted disease clinics. Among the factors affecting condom use are negative attitudes toward condoms. People tend not to use condoms if they believe that condoms compromise the pleasure of intercourse, that condoms are unnatural, and that one's partner is likely to be offended if condoms are introduced (Marvin & Steinmetz, 1987; Siegel & Gibson, 1988).

Watters (1988), who conducted in-depth interviews with 27 injection drug users in San Francisco's inner-city areas, found that most of the men interviewed disliked condoms. Many of the women had sex without condoms because their sexual partners did not want to use them. The women who were engaged in prostitution would often waive condom use if it meant keeping a customer.

Wermuth's (Wermuth, Ham, & Hester, 1989) survey of 77 women sexual partners of injection drug users found strong negative reactions to suggesting condom use by their male partners. The survey asked study participants, "What do you think your partner's reaction would be if you suggested that he always use a condom?" Responses included reports of, or expectations of, partners' anger and violence (30%), refusals to wear condoms (39%), and responses that "You're crazy" to suggest condom use (10%). In addition, individual women reported responses such as their male partners' ending the relationship or throwing away or ripping up condoms to prevent their use.

Negative dispositions toward condom use among men, and ambivalence on the part of some women, discourage the use of condoms (Wermuth et al., 1991). In an analysis of Wermuth's data, male partners' negative attitudes toward condoms were found to decrease condom use among female sexual partners of injection drug users (Choi, Wermuth, & Sorensen, 1990).

Economic and Emotional Dependence

The model of individual risk reduction based on health beliefs assumes that, when faced with a noncompliant partner, the highly motivated individual chooses not to engage in risky sexual activity. Assumptions of individually driven decision making may be more valid for casual encounters in which there are no fears of reprisals or other serious costs for refused sex. When individuals do not have equal "bargaining power" in relationships, however, this assumption may not apply (Collins, 1975; Worth, 1989). Especially in longer-term and marital relationships, in which there is greater personal investment, individuals often weigh the possible loss of the relationship that pressing for condom use could bring. Des Jarlais and Friedman (1988) noted that such emotional commitment would make it more difficult for injection drug users to negotiate condom use in steady relationships than in casual sexual encounters.

Economic and emotional dependence is the most salient barrier to risk reduction among women partners of injection drug users (Peterson & Marin, 1988; M. T. Fullilove et al., 1990b; Worth, 1989). Poor women are constrained in their choices about relationships and living situations, and they may not experience the freedom to regulate sexual practices or to separate themselves from men who put them at risk for AIDS. Concerns regarding food, shelter, and care of their children may overshadow worries about AIDS (Mays & Cochran, 1988). Needs for emotional intimacy with a man may add to the difficulty of altering sexual behavior. Outsiders who advocate abstinence or condom use may be looked upon as threatening to a woman's survival. If her drug use and sexual behavior bring her economic and emotional support from a partner, it could be difficult for a woman to exchange these circumstances for financial and personal uncertainties.

The Need for Partner Communication and Cooperation

Research on correlates of contraceptive use among married couples has shown that verbal, empathetic, and concurrent communication increases the use of birth control methods (Marvin & Steinmetz, 1987). Similarly, the following two studies suggest that condom use among injection drug users requires communication and cooperation between sexual partners. Magura et al.'s (1990) study of 211 methadone patients in New York City found that condom use was associated with greater personal acceptance of condoms and greater partner receptivity to sexual protection. The Partners Outreach Project data (*n* = 73) also showed discussion of condom use and the man's positive condom attitudes as predictors of condom use among women sexual partners of injection drug users (Choi et al., 1990).

Cultural values affect communication and cooperation between sexual partners. When a premium is placed on male prerogatives in sexual relationships, women's choices and abilities to initiate discussion and changes are hampered. Especially among less acculturated Hispanic couples, for example, it is not acceptable for women to bring up the topic of sexual relations or to propose practices such as using condoms. Consequently, it is problematic for women to be assertive in protecting themselves from possible HIV infection. When condom use is initiated by women it has been reported to provoke distrust, violence, and abandonment (Mays & Cochran, 1988; Wermuth et al., 1991).

AIDS Stigma and Denial

The AIDS epidemic has stirred strong negative public reactions to persons infected with HIV. The general public has expressed fear and hostility toward HIV-infected individuals. Some business communities have discriminated against those persons in their jobs and in insurance coverage. Until recently, government officials have been reluctant to fund widespread public educational programs that included safe sex guidelines for AIDS prevention (Panem, 1987).

The major sources of AIDS stigma have been the lethal nature of the disease and the prevalence of HIV infection among marginalized groups (Herek & Glunt, 1988). AIDS has been perceived as an illness that is life-threatening and can be transmitted by specific behaviors. It has also been believed to be the disease of gay men and injection drug users. The notion of AIDS patients' promiscuity has resulted in blaming victims for the cause of their condition. The pre-existing prejudice toward gay men and injection drug users has resulted in a double stigma.

Social disapproval of illicit drug use and promiscuity has caused many injection drug users to deny their risk for AIDS and has hampered them from seeking HIV antibody testing and early treatment (Herek & Glunt, 1988; Siegel & Gibson, 1988). Injection drug users, who are accustomed to taking risks, are likely to deny that their sexual or drug use behavior could be dangerous, especially if they feel unable to change their risky practices. Women sexual partners of injection drug users are often secretive about their partners' drug use because injection drug use and relationships with "addicts" are stigmatized. They deny their risk for AIDS and isolate themselves from those who could encourage them to take protective measures.

PUBLIC HEALTH IMPLICATIONS AND FUTURE RESEARCH

The health belief model suggests that if we raise the threat of infection, increase response and self-efficacy, and improve communications, people can be helped to change their attitudes toward the threat and reduce risky behavior. This model has become a guiding principle in designing AIDS prevention programs such as mass media campaigns, flyers with AIDS prevention messages, and individual and group counseling.

Despite a variety of AIDS prevention efforts, many injection drug users and their sexual partners are still practicing unsafe sex. The foregoing discussion about barriers to risk reduction indicates that AIDS prevention programs need to include couple-oriented approaches and expansion of drug treatment. The finding that discussion is a predictor of condom use, in particular, suggests that AIDS prevention models based on individualistic conceptions may be inadequate to address the problem of sexual transmission of HIV in the drug-injecting population. Since condom use involves negotiations about changes in sexual practices and requires the cooperation of both sexual partners, couples and their relationship issues need to be included in our prevention efforts. In addition, because the data show that heavy drug users and those with low self-efficacy tend not to practice safer sex, expanded drug treatment efforts, individual and group counseling, and promotion of self-help among injection drug users must play a central role in AIDS prevention by helping them with their addiction and other emotional problems.

AIDS prevention efforts should take special care to involve ethnic minority groups, given their cultural differences and socioeconomic vulnerability. AIDS educational materials should contain culturally sensitive messages about safer sex. For example, the condom campaign among Hispanic male injection drug users might emphasize that the man should take some responsibility for protecting the family from the AIDS threat, since Hispanic cultures promote the importance of the family and machismo (Peterson & Marin, 1988). For dissemination of AIDS-related information, more appropriate mediums should be used. In the African-American community, television, billboard, and ethnic magazines and newspapers may be more effective in influencing attitudes and perceptions about AIDS (Mays, 1989). Hispanic communities may benefit from media campaigns aired by Spanish radio and television stations (Amaro, 1988).

To insure the success of massive preventive campaigns and outreach programs, it is essential to seek to involve community leaders and ethnic organizations. Historically, minority groups have relied on their communities for their survival. In turn, the communities have exerted great influence in shaping norms, attitudes, and behaviors among their members. To gain community cooperation and access to social networks of drug users, Mata and Jorquez (1989) suggest that minority health educators be recruited who have credibility and respect among injection drug users and official legitimacy among community health professionals.

Finally, drug treatment centers should offer AIDS education and counseling to their minority clients. Drug treatment provides an important opportunity to expose minority injection drug users to AIDS educational materials and counseling services designed for AIDS risk behavior (Peterson & Marin, 1988; Mata & Jorquez, 1989). To better serve minority populations, drug treatment clinics should recruit ethnic minority staff members who understand the cultural values and concerns of minority drug users. Since some minority health workers at first may not be prepared to provide AIDS counseling, special attention should be paid to their in-service trainings (Peterson & Marin, 1988).

Analysis of risk behaviors is a first step toward understanding the very complex and sensitive issue of sexual behavior and AIDS prevention. There are several areas that future research should address. The efficacy of the health belief model requires further empirical tests. Most research has focused on the direct effect of health beliefs on behavioral outcomes, although the model suggests their indirect role in risk reduction. Future research should examine, for example, whether AIDS prevention increases individuals' self-efficacy, and in turn, whether improved self-efficacy helps to modify behavior. Moreover, the adequacy of the health belief model as an AIDS prevention guideline for the drug injection population should be addressed, to investigate the relative influence of health beliefs in relation to psychological and socioeconomic difficulties experienced by injection drug users and their sexual partners. Furthermore, since ethnic minority groups are overrepresented in the drug-injecting population at risk for AIDS, cross-cultural studies of sexual behavior should be conducted to increase our understanding and sensitivity. Finally, the evaluation of existing interventions should contribute to the development of more adequate and innovative AIDS prevention programs for injection drug users and their sexual partners.

Chapter 5

Theoretical Background

DAVID R. GIBSON
JOSEPH A. CATANIA
JOHN L. PETERSON

Transmission of HIV occurs when people share body fluids during sex or when they inject drugs. Because such behaviors are partly under the control of conscious processes, they are potentially modifiable. It is far from clear, however, how that potential can be realized. Simply informing people of the risks of certain behaviors has generally not proven to be effective. Many injection drug users, for example, continue to share injection equipment, despite the fact that nearly all are aware of the danger of this practice (Selwyn, Feiner, Cox, Lipshutz, & Cohen, 1987). Like certain high-risk sexual behaviors, sharing of infected needles is a behavior that has been highly resistant to change, although significant behavior change appears to have occurred in several U.S. cities (see Chapter 3).

If information is not enough to change behavior, what is? In this chapter, to help answer this question, we turn to literature on health psychology. Health psychology is a branch of applied psychology that is concerned with understanding and changing behaviors affecting personal health (Stone, Cohen, & Adler, 1979). One approach has been to identify psychological and social correlates of behaviors that promote or endanger health; these correlates, it is thought, can help to inform efforts to change behavior. Here we consider a number of health psychology concepts that have important implications for HIV-related behaviors. The framework we employ is the AIDS Risk Reduction Model (ARRM), an eclectic model integrating elements of prior models, including the classic Health Belief Model (Becker, 1974; Janz & Becker, 1984), decision-making theory (Fishbein & Azjen, 1975; Gross & McMullen, 1983), self-efficacy theory (Bandura, 1977), and theories of interpersonal processes and the role of emotions in behavior (Janis, 1967; Rogers, 1983). The ARRM is useful as a model not only for organizing these concepts, but also for understanding their role in the process of behavior change. After a brief overview of the ARRM, we discuss a number of its constituent variables and review the empirical evidence of the part they play in HIV-related behavior. Finally, we consider high-risk behaviors within a broader social context, examining specifically the role of gender and race/ethnicity.

Early efforts to understand health behaviors focused on the effect of fear appeals (e.g., Janis, 1967). It was thought, for example, that showing people graphic photographs of diseased lungs might encourage them to quit smoking or deter them from becoming smokers. We now know that behavior change involves many other variables, some of which have to do more with common sense than with fear. The health belief model (Becker, 1974) suggested that in making decisions affecting health, people weigh the costs and benefits of different health practices. The health belief model views health behaviors as a function of people's perceived susceptibility and perceived severity of a health condition, and the perceived benefits and barriers to behavior change. The model has been embraced more widely by health educators than by academic psychologists, who have pointed to the role of other important variables, such as self-efficacy (see, e.g., Bandura, 1977). In this context, "self-efficacy" refers to a person's perceived ability to implement recommended health practices. Exogenous to models of health behaviors, of course, are sociocultural variables such as class and gender. Sociocultural variables may exert their influence on behavior via health beliefs, but also in more direct ways.

The health belief model and related models have proven to be useful tools for understanding preventive health behaviors. Beliefs about susceptibility to heart disease, cancer, and tuberculosis, and about the benefits of identifying these conditions, all predict subsequent voluntary checkups (Haefner & Kirscht, 1970). Similarly, in regression analyses, beliefs about susceptibility, severity, and benefits explain much of the variance in willingness to be vaccinated for influenza and hepatitis (Bodenheimer, Fulton, & Kramer, 1986). Empirical findings such as these are helpful in identifying positive and negative correlates of health-related behaviors, which can inform health educators in designing interventions to help people to adopt these behaviors.

THE AIDS RISK REDUCTION MODEL

In this chapter we focus on health psychology principles with implications for the design of preventive interventions with drug users and their sexual partners. A small but growing body of literature has examined correlates of HIV-related high-risk behavior among gay and bisexual men, and a handful of studies have looked at predictors of high-risk practices of adolescents and adult heterosexuals (for a review, see Catania, Kegeles, & Coates, 1990). As yet there is little evidence concerning the role of psychosocial variables in drug-related behaviors. To help fill this gap, we draw on our own and others' unpublished data. Chapter 4 discusses the correlates of high-risk sexual practices among injection drug users and their sexual partners. Because of the wide array of high-risk practices and methods for assessing them, the findings are often inconsistent (Catania et al., 1990; Kirscht & Joseph, 1989).

Nearly all work to date has focused on relationships between predictor variables and levels of risk behaviors or changes in behaviors over time. Catania et al. (1990) point out that this approach misses the role that different psychosocial variables play at different stages in the change process. For example, AIDS knowledge may be important in assessing personal risk, whereas self-efficacy beliefs come into play only after a person has committed himself or herself to risk reduction. Catania and his colleagues have proposed a three-stage model, the ARRM, to describe people's efforts to change sexual behaviors related to HIV transmission. Although the focus of the model is on sexual behavior, Catania et al. argue that with minor modifications the model can be applied to other HIV-related behaviors, including those of injection drug users.

The ARRM is not intended to be the last word on HIV-related behavior. Instead, its authors view it as a heuristic device for integrating a wide variety of concepts derived from diverse theoretical perspectives. As empirical findings accumulate, the model may have to be modified significantly.

The elements of the model are pictured in Table 5.l. According to the model, behavior change is accompanied by successive stages of labeling, commitment, and action. At the labeling stage (Stage 1), a person learns how AIDS is transmitted and becomes aware of his or her susceptibility to disease. Knowledge and susceptibility together prompt people to ask whether their behavior puts them at risk. At the commitment stage (Stage 2), a person discovers effective ways of reducing risk (in health psychology terms, develops response efficacy) and begins to develop self-efficacy in coping with the threat. Response efficacy and self-efficacy help to build the person's confidence or expectancy that he or she can implement behavioral changes. Finally, at the enactment stage (Stage 3), a person begins to take concrete steps toward the goal of behavior change, through either self-help or seeking help from others. Talking with and seeking help from others, such as sexual partners, increase the odds of success. As noted in Table 5.1, aversive emotions

TABLE 5.1. AIDS Risk Reduction Model (ARRM): Influences

Stage	Some [hypothesized] influences	Outcome indicators
1. Labeling	Transmission knowledge Susceptibility Aversive emotions Social influences[a]	Is your behavior putting you at risk for HIV infection?
2. Commitment	Aversive emotions Perceived benefits of making changes (response efficacy) Self-efficacy Social influences[a]	Do you expect to do "*x*" in the next 4 weeks?
3. Enactment	Aversive emotions Communications skill Social influences[a]	What have you done?

Note. Adapted from "Toward an Understanding of Risk Behavior: An AIDS Risk-Reduction Model" by J. A. Catania, S. Kegeles, and T. J. Coates, 1990, *Health Education Quarterly*, *17*, 53–92. Copyright 1990 by SOPHE. Adapted by permission.
[a]Social support, norms.

(such as persistent anxiety about being at risk) come into play at all stages of the process of behavioral changes. Likewise, social influences (the influence of friends, peers, and "significant others") are important at all stages to the extent that they provide cues about a person's susceptibility to infection or reminders of commitment to change (Catania et al., 1990).

In discussing the application of the ARRM to HIV-related behaviors, we draw here on a small but growing number of studies, mostly of gay men, that have examined correlates of high-risk sexual behavior. Unfortunately, there are very few data on the antecedents of injection drug users' high-risk practices. Chapter 4 discusses relevant information with regard to injection drug users' sexual behaviors. In this chapter we review the scanty evidence (mostly unpublished data of our own) that exists on injection drug users' HIV-related drug-taking practices. The data are from a San Francisco drug treatment sample.

The data from the sample were gathered in face-to-face interviews with 226 heroin addicts in heroin detoxification treatment program at San Francisco General Hospital conducted between December 1987 and May 1989. The demographic and treatment characteristics of the sample appear in Table 5.2. Respondents were paid $10 for a 20-minute interview, which elicited information about demographic characteristics, AIDS knowledge, attitudes and beliefs about AIDS risk, and

TABLE 5.2 Demographic Characteristics and Needle-Sharing Practices of Sample ($N = 226$)

Characteristics	Percent
Age	
Under 30	15
30–39	47
40 and over	38
Gender	
Male	67
Female	33
Race/ethnicity	
Black	35
Latin	20
White	39
Other	6
Shared a "dirty" needle in the last month	
Not at all	68
1–5 times	13
6 or more time	20

self-reported sexual and injection-drug-related behaviors. The attitude and beliefs assessed included AIDS anxiety, susceptibility, acceptance of guidelines to reduce risk (response efficacy), and self-reported self-efficacy and communication skill in negotiating low-risk behavior. Details concerning the construction of the knowledge and attitude scales are reported elsewhere (Gibson, Choi, Catania, Sorensen, & Kegeles, 1991).

High-risk behavior is connected not only with attitudes and beliefs (both of drug users and of their peers), but also with situational factors. Ethnographic studies suggest that needle sharing is associated with attendance at shooting galleries and lack of resources for purchasing sterile needles (Des Jarlais, Friedman, & Strug, 1986; S. Murphy, 1987). Needle sharing appears to be related to the difficulty drug users have in obtaining sterile injection equipment and the inability to purchase sterile needles, as well as to the injecting of drugs in "shooting galleries" or other public places (Magura et al., 1989b; Gibson et al., 1991). Situational factors, of course, both reflect and contribute to HIV-related attitudes and beliefs. Drug users who frequent shooting galleries, for example, probably will not report much self-efficacy.

In the remainder of this chapter, we review evidence concerning the role that health beliefs play in high-risk behavior. In addition, we consider whether there might be more straightforward explanations for behavior—for example, whether needle sharing might be simply explained by lack of access to sterile needles. We also examine social and cultural variations in health beliefs that may have implications for preventive interventions.

HIV-RELATED KNOWLEDGE, ATTITUDES, AND BELIEFS

Knowledge

According to the authors of the ARRM, knowledge comes into play at the first stage of behavior change, at a point where a drug user might perceive problems with his or her behavior. Knowledge about HIV infection runs the gamut from basic facts that almost everyone knows (e.g., that AIDS can be transmitted sexually) to what a colleague has referred to as "AIDS trivia." In our work with injection drug users, we have tried to provide only essential information, facts that injection drug users must know in order to accurately assess their personal level of risk. Knowledge about routes of transmission of the virus, for example, is essential for evaluating whether one's behaviors are risky. Once a person has determined that he or she may be at risk, information about coping with specific problems may also be helpful. Accurate, relevant information about antibody testing, syringe exchanges, and proper procedures for using condoms may facilitate the adoption of low-risk practices.

Empirical findings on the relationship between knowledge and HIV risk behaviors are mixed. Cross-sectional and longitudinal studies of gay men show that knowledge about HIV transmission and "safe sex" guidelines predict high-risk sexual behavior (such as unprotected anal intercourse and number of sexual partners), as well as the reduction of such behaviors over time (Emmons et al., 1986; Kegeles, Catania, Coates, & Adler, 1986; McKusick, Coates, Wiley, Morin, & Stall, 1987). Among heterosexual college students, knowledge is related to numbers of sexual partners but not to frequency of condom use (Baldwin & Baldwin, 1988). Other cross-sectional and longitudinal studies of gay men have found no relationship between knowledge and high-risk sexual practices.

Catania et al. (1990), among others, argue that knowledge is important only at the early stage in a change process; it is a necessary but not a sufficient cause of behavior change. Data from our San Francisco drug treatment sample indicate that nearly all drug users had the essential facts concerning risk education. When asked to name different strategies for reducing sex- and drug-related risk, nearly all drug users mentioned quitting drugs, not sharing needles, and sterilizing syringes as effective. Similarly, most identified abstinence, monogamy, and condoms as effective ways of reducing sexual risk. In our sample, knowledge at this most basic level appears to have been more of a constant than a variable.

Susceptibility

Like knowledge, susceptibility is important at the early stages of the change process, when a drug user first perceives that there may be problems with his or her behavior. Susceptibility figured prominently in the original health belief model, along with perceived severity and perceived benefits and barriers to behavior change (Janz & Becker, 1984). Susceptibility is not synonymous with knowledge about how HIV is transmitted, since some people who are aware of how it is transmitted nevertheless do not perceive themselves at risk (Coates, Morin, Lo, Stall, & McKusick, 1987). Denial may play some part in this, perhaps supported by confusion about whether the body's immune response is protective. Without unambiguous symptoms, drug users may downplay their vulnerability. A complicating factor is that many of the early symptoms of HIV infection (flu-like infections, night sweats, etc.) are also symptoms of heroin withdrawal. Recognition of susceptibility may therefore be delayed.

Empirical findings suggest that susceptibility is an important variable. For example, when knowledge is held constant, susceptibility predicts reduction in high-risk sexual behaviors, number of sex partners, and avoidance of anonymous sex among gay men (Emmons et al., 1986; Kegeles et al., 1986). However, Emmons et al. found no relationship between susceptibility and frequency of anal intercourse, and longitudinal analyses have not found susceptibility to be related to number of sex partners and anonymous sex (Joseph et al., 1987).

Catania et al. (1990) have suggested that the relationship between susceptibility and high-risk practices may be reciprocal. Injection drug users, for example, may report being susceptible because they have shared needles with other drug users. At the same time, a feeling of susceptibility may prompt them to do fewer risky things. Longitudinal data are needed to permit us to examine these reciprocal influences. In our own cross-sectional data, susceptibility was positively correlated (.22) with needle sharing. (In a logistic regression that included other health beliefs, however, susceptibility did not account for significant unique variance.)

Response Efficacy

"Response efficacy" refers to the perceived effectiveness of recommended health practices (Bandura, 1977; Rogers, 1975; cf. the concept of "perceived benefit" in literature on the health belief model—Becker, 1974). Response efficacy comes into play at Stage 2 (commitment) of the ARRM. At this stage, having acknowledged problematic behavior, a drug user may take the additional step of making a commitment to risk reduction. He or she may then begin to consider actions that promise to reduce the risk of contracting HIV. For example, drug treatment may be contemplated as an option. Or the drug user may resolve to shoot drugs only at home, where a supply of sterile needles can be kept, and where running water and disinfectant bleach can be used to clean injection equipment. Commitment to making such positive steps, however, will depend on the drug user's perception of their effectiveness.

Response efficacy appears to be involved in decisions to make behavioral change, and, under conditions of self-efficacy, to result in actual behavioral change (Strecher, DeVellis, Becker, & Rosenstock, 1986; Wurtele & Maddux, 1987). Response efficacy has also been implicated in behaviors related to transmission of HIV, although again the findings are contradictory. In three studies of gay men, acceptance of safe sex guidelines was negatively associated both cross-sectionally and longitudinally with high-risk behavior (Emmons et al., 1986; Kegeles et al., 1986; McKusick, Horstman, & Coates, 1985b). In another study, however, also of gay men, there appeared to be no relationship between response efficacy and high-risk sexual practices (Joseph et al., 1987).

Our own data from San Francisco suggest that response efficacy plays little role in risk reduction, perhaps because the drug users we interviewed were persuaded of recommendations concerning reduction of risk. In San Francisco, prevention campaigns have greatly raised the level of awareness of AIDS among injection drug users.

Self-Efficacy

"Self-efficacy" is a key construct in literature on health psychology. The term refers to a person's perceived ability to implement recommended health practices. In relation to HIV, self-efficacy is critical to development of commitment to risk reduction (Stage 2 of the ARRM model). A drug user lacking confidence in his or her capacity to make behavioral changes is unlikely to make good on that commitment. Self-efficacy is particularly important in situations where one is sorely tempted to do things that nevertheless endanger one's health. An example would be an injection drug user who is experiencing severe withdrawal. Lacking self-efficacy, he or she may yield to the need to relieve withdrawal symptoms (particularly craving for drugs) and disregard his or her better judgment about not sharing or sterilizing needles.

Self-efficacy may also be important when it comes to enacting risk reduction (Stage 3 of the ARRM model). Behavior change is not a gestalt switch. Rather, it is typically a process of gradually incorporating new behaviors into, and eliminating old ones from, one's repertoire. Relapse to unsafe practices is to be expected. The greater a person's self-efficacy, however, the greater the likelihood that he or she will return to safe practices. Marlatt and George (1989) believe that this element of resiliency is essential for long-term behavior change.

Numerous studies have documented self-efficacy's importance in the performance of a wide variety of health-promoting behaviors (for a review, see Beck & Frankel, 1981). Not surprisingly, there is also evidence that it is important in HIV risk reduction. In two studies of gay men, self-efficacy predicted low-risk sexual behavior both cross-sectionally and longitudinally (McKusick et al., 1985b, 1987).

Self-efficacy is also associated with increased condom use in heterosexual injection drug users undergoing heroin detoxification treatment. In our own data (Sample A), self-efficacy was highly and negatively correlated (-.47) with self-reported needle sharing.

Communication Skill

Although it has not been given wide attention in the health psychology literature, communication skill may be important where others are involved in behaviors affecting personal health. In such cases, the ability to engage others in discussion of the behaviors in question may be critical. Sexual practices, of course, are one large class of such behaviors. Sexual communications have been linked in several studies to success in changing sexual behaviors, including the introduction of condoms into a sexual relationship (Schinke, Gilchrist, & Small, 1979; Polit-O'Hara & Kahn, 1985). Data from our own group concerning the role of communication skill in negotiating condom use among injection drug users are discussed in Chapter 4. In our sample, communication skill in negotiating safe injection practices was correlated negatively (-.32) with self-reported needle sharing. Communication skill and self-efficacy were highly correlated (.55), suggesting that the ability to arrange safe practices may be integral to perceived efficacy.

Social Support

A variable closely related to communication skill is social support. In the context of personal health, "social support" may be defined as emotional and instrumental assistance that a person can call on in making behavioral changes. Although findings are somewhat contradictory, social support is associated with many positive health behaviors (Cleary et al., 1986; House, 1981; Nathanson & Becker, 1986), including reduction of high-risk sexual practices (Emmons et al., 1986; Joseph et al., 1987; Richardson, Schott, McGuigan, & Levine, 1987; Stall, Ekstrand, Pollack, McKusick, & Coates, 1990b).

With reference to HIV risk reduction, social support is probably most important at the enactment stage of risk reduction (Stage 3 of the ARRM). Studies of gay men show that seropositive gay men who have the support of a primary sexual partner or who can call on help from friends are more likely to reduce their frequency of unprotected anal intercourse (Catania, Kegeles, & Coates, 1988). In our own data, support of one's sexual partner was correlated .26 with the use of condoms.

Other Variables

Our discussion of HIV-related attitudes is by no means exhaustive. Our intention has been to introduce some key health concepts relevant to transmission with HIV. The potential role of such concepts in HIV risk reduction needs to be carefully considered in the design of interventions to help drug users cope with the threat of infection.

Among the variables we have not considered at length are perceived severity and (AIDS-specific) anxiety. Perceived severity was a key variable in the original health belief model, although to our knowledge no one has examined its relationship to HIV-related behavior. In our work with injection drug users, we have not given it much attention, on the assumption that drug users uniformly view AIDS as a severe and lethal medical condition. Whether this assumption always holds true can be debated. In San Francisco, relatively few drug users personally know someone who has contracted the disease, although as many as 20% of San Francisco drug users are believed to be infected with HIV. When asked to name the two most common infections that AIDS patients get, fewer than a third in 1988–1989 were able to identify these as (pneumocystis) pneumonia and skin cancer (Kaposi's sarcoma). A clear understanding of the seriousness of the disease may help to bring home the importance of risk reduction.

Although our data include a measure of AIDS anxiety, we have not discussed anxiety at length because of its close association with susceptibility (the two were correlated .50 in our sample). Catania et al. (1990) suggest that anxiety may play a role in movement from one stage to the next of the change process. Although high levels of anxiety may lead to denial of a threat (Leventhal, Zimmerman, & Gutmann, 1984), moderate levels may strengthen commitment to make changes. In cross-sectional data from our sample, however, anxiety was positively associated (.17) with needle sharing.

SOCIOCULTURAL INFLUENCES ON HIGH-RISK BEHAVIOR

As noted earlier, the ARRM is derived from an eclectic array of prior models, including those of decision-making theory, the classic health belief model, self-efficacy theory, and theories of emotional states and interpersonal processes (Catania et al., 1990). The focus of the ARRM is on psychological and cognitive variables that lead to labeling of high-risk behaviors as problematic, to development of commitment to changing those behaviors, and to subsequent seeking and enactment of solutions directed at reducing high-risk behaviors.

Like the models on which it is based, the ARRM emphasizes the role of the individual's perceptions more than objective reality, although it incorporates both social norms and support and help that the individual may receive from others. It is possible, however, to imagine other situational or structural factors that may impinge on behavior. Huang, Watters, and Case (1989), for example, found no relationship between needle hygiene (use of bleach for disinfecting syringes) and perceived susceptibility, response efficacy, or self-efficacy, but did find that hygiene was associated with "ecological" factors such as the availability of cleaning reagents.

In a simultaneous logistic regression of data gathered from our drug treatment sample (Gibson et al., 1991) we examined the impact on needle sharing of many constituent variables of the ARRM (including susceptibility, AIDS anxiety, response efficacy, self-efficacy, and communication skill), along with sociodemographic characteristics and situational or "ecological" variables (e.g., whether drugs were injected in a shooting gallery or other public places).

Needle sharing was strongly related to shooting drugs in a shooting gallery or other public place (odds ratio of 2.65; that is, drug users shooting in a public place were more than 2 1/2 times more likely to share), but was also strongly predicted by self-efficacy (odds ratio of 0.48 for each point on a 5-point scale). Of some interest is the finding that self-efficacy and injection of drugs in a public place were correlated -.31, suggesting that health beliefs and situational factors may be related. The number of sterile needles used in the past 30 days was negatively related to needle sharing (odds ratio of 0.89 for each 10 such needles used).

Over 80% of AIDS cases among injection drug users and cases of AIDS among women are among nonwhites (Selik, Castro, & Pappaioanou, 1988). The preponderance of AIDS cases among nonwhites, however, cannot be attributed solely to the high proportion of injection drug users who are minority group members. Other sociocultural factors therefore need to be examined to account for racial/ethnic differences in high-risk practices. As earlier noted, sociocultural variables may be considered exogenous to the ARRM; ARRM variables may or may not mediate much of their impact. Stated differently, relationships among model variables may differ greatly, depending on one's membership in different sociocultural groups. For example, evidence presented in Chapters 4 and 9 indicates that there may be a much weaker relationship between self-efficacy and adherence to safe sex guidelines for women than for men, since women may exert less control in heterosexual relationships.

Research by Catania and his colleagues (Catania, McDermott, & Wood, 1984) suggests that in terms of traditional sexual roles, men are more likely to initiate sexual intercourse, although women share in decisions about sexual practices. Concerning the role of race/ethnicity, it has been suggested that nonwhite addicts may have greater difficulty in obtaining new needles and syringes because of the cost and legal restrictions on the supply of sterile equipment (Drucker, 1986; Friedland et al., 1986; Marmor, Des Jarlais, Friedman, Lyden, & El-Sadr, 1984). According to this view, economic disadvantages might weaken relationships between, for example, AIDS knowledge and behavior.

In fact, as Chapter 3 explains, the disproportionately high rates of AIDS and HIV infection among African-Americans and Hispanics are not consistently accounted for by needle sharing (Brown, Murphy, & Primm, 1987; Lewis & Watters, 1988; Magura et al., 1989b; Guydish, Abramowitz, Woods, Black, & Sorensen, 1990a). Our own data indicate that white drug injectors in the sample were more than twice as likely as nonwhite injectors to report sharing a "dirty" needle in the 30 days prior to the interview (odds ratio of 2.55). Why? An examination of correlates of white race reveals that white drug users were more likely to shoot drugs in a shooting gallery or other public place (r = .25). Whites did not differ from nonwhites, however, in health beliefs, which were uncorrelated with white race. African-Americans were less likely to share needles (zero-order correlation = -.31). Why? They were also less likely (-.31) to shoot in public, and had higher levels of self-efficacy (r = .26) and communication skill (r = .14). Moreover, they had lower levels of susceptibility (-.18) anxiety (-.17), perhaps reflecting lower levels of needle sharing. The moral is that models such as the ARRM may tell us quite different things, depending on which social group we are dealing with. In designing interventions, we need to pay careful to the special needs of different populations.

IMPLICATIONS

Chapters 6 through 9 consider the implications of health psychology principles for the design of preventive interventions. A few comments, however, are in order here. First, different interventions may be appropriate at different stages of the AIDS epidemic. At the early stages, information may be critical for raising drug users' awareness of the nature of the threat. At this stage of the epidemic, billboards, television spots, and educational leaflets may be the most appropriate way of reaching a large audience. Institutional and grassroots efforts also need to be initiated by those people who have contact with drug users in drug treatment programs, as do outreach efforts with drug users on the street. Without basic information about how they are at risk, drug users cannot begin to make needed changes in their behavior.

A second point is that information is necessary but not sufficient to change behavior. We have seen that self-efficacy apparently plays an important role in risk reduction, and that it is strongly correlated with communication skill. Both variables are important at the level of developing commitment to behavior change. Neither is likely to be much influenced by distribution of leaflets or messages in the mass media. Clinical interventions such as those described in the next four chapters may be needed to build drug users' and sexual partners' self-confidence to the point that they can resist needle sharing and other high-risk practices. Interventions, however, need to be cost-effective and capable of reaching significant numbers of those at risk.

Part 2

PREVENTIVE INTERVENTIONS WITH DRUG USERS AND THEIR SEXUAL PARTNERS

Chapter 6

Drug Abuse Treatment for HIV-Infected Patients

STEVEN L. BATKI
JULIE LONDON

Substance abuse treatment is becoming an important AIDS prevention strategy as the AIDS epidemic spreads among injection drug users. Although AIDS prevention campaigns can be effectively disseminated outside drug abuse programs (Watters, 1987), prevention efforts may be more comprehensive, intensive, and accessible if conducted in the setting of substance abuse treatment. With the increase in HIV-infected injection drug users, treatment programs are admitting patients with complex clinical presentations. These clinical problems challenge the capabilities of traditional drug abuse treatment models to address the special needs of HIV-infected addicts (Batki, Sorensen, Gibson, & Maude-Griffin, 1990c). Both AIDS and the recent cocaine epidemic among injection drug users are making it necessary for treatment providers to develop and integrate a wider range of clinical services. Drug abuse treatment facilities that admit large numbers of seropositive injection drug users may have to modify their "recovery-oriented" treatment philosophies (Sorensen, Costantini, & London, 1989b) and change treatment approaches and administrative policies as a result of the AIDS and cocaine crises. This chapter examines how clinical interventions in the setting of substance abuse treatment can prevent the spread of AIDS.

A number of different clinical approaches are being developed in response to the need for preventing and treating HIV among this population. This chapter begins with a discussion of why drug abuse treatment is AIDS prevention, and an overview of traditional models of drug abuse treatment. This is followed by a description of opiate addiction and of how methadone maintenance treatment (MMT) can be a useful setting for providing HIV-infected injection drug users with comprehensive treatment services. Treatment outcome for opiate and stimulant abuse among HIV-infected patients in MMT is reviewed. A subsequent section focuses on the primary medical care that HIV-infected opiate addicts require while in outpatient drug abuse treatment, and describes our experience in conducting and evaluating an on-site medical clinic at San Francisco General Hospital (SFGH) Substance Abuse Services. Psychiatric and psychosocial problems of seropositive injection drug users, as well as a framework for managing their mental health problems, are presented next. The special problems of providing AIDS prevention services to ethnic and sexual minority injection drug users are also discussed. The final section takes stock of the clinical interventions reviewed and provides recommendations for future clinical services and research.

Some of the points subsequently discussed in this chapter are prefaced in an illustrative manner by several brief vignettes describing the treatment of a patient, Mary.

Mary: Admission to Treatment

Mary is a 39-year-old woman who has come to SFGH Substance Abuse Services asking for admission to MMT. She has been a heroin addict for over 20 years. There are few openings available in the MMT program, but she is admitted readily, along with her common-law husband. The reason Mary and her husband are admitted so quickly is that she has recently tested positive for HIV antibody, and the program to which she has applied has a policy of preferentially admitting patients with HIV infection.

DRUG ABUSE TREATMENT: CLINICAL INTERVENTIONS AND AIDS PREVENTION

Drug abuse treatment is essential for HIV-infected injection drug users for several reasons. First, and perhaps most important, drug abuse treatment for injection drug users is a form of AIDS prevention. Prevention occurs when needle use and needle sharing are reduced through the decrease in drug use brought about by such treatments as MMT (Ball, Lange, Myers, & Friedman, 1988). Prevention may also be an indirect outcome of the reduction of impulsive, unsafe sex acts associated with intoxicated, disinhibited states or with sex-for-drugs transactions (R. E. Fullilove, Fullilove, Bowser, & Gross, 1990a).

Drug use can create a pressured and impulsive lifestyle that does not encourage appropriate concern for safety, either in sexual behavior or in the hygiene of drug use itself. Drug use may also be a cofactor for

HIV by lowering resistance to the virus through impairing cell-mediated immunity. Drugs that have been implicated in immune suppression include the opiates, cocaine, alcohol, marijuana, and others (MacGregor, 1987). Once infected with HIV, drug users may be at added risk for developing many forms of morbidity associated with HIV. Continued parenteral drug use may stimulate HIV activation and replication (Zagury et al., 1986), and also places users at risk for developing secondary infections. Finally, psychopathology associated with drug use may worsen the neuropsychiatric and mental health problems associated with AIDS itself.

Reducing drug use through treatment can be expected to reduce a number of the above-listed risks for AIDS. Moreover, drug abuse treatment is important because it provides a setting for delivering other services needed by HIV-infected patients. These services include psychiatric care, medical care, social services, and AIDS education. Drug abuse treatment may also be helpful in reducing the morbidity associated with HIV infection, probably through lessening the assaults on the immune system and decreasing exposure to infectious agents (Des Jarlais et al., 1987b).

TYPES OF DRUG ABUSE TREATMENT

Drug abuse treatment programs can be broadly categorized as belonging to one of three basic modalities: self-help, residential treatment, and outpatient treatment. Treatment of HIV-infected patients in any of these modalities presents a number of problems as well as opportunities, and requires the use of novel strategies.

Self-Help Programs

Examples of self-help programs are the "Twelve-Step" groups such as Alcoholics Anonymous (AA) and other programs modeled after AA but designed for other forms of substance abuse, such as Cocaine Anonymous (CA) and Narcotics Anonymous (NA) (Nichols, 1988; Nurco, Wegner, Stephenson, Makofsky, & Shaffer, 1983). NA may be of particular importance for HIV-infected drug users, because many participants are former injection drug users themselves, who can offer peer support, identification, and therapeutic confrontation. Self-help groups probably offer the most widely accessible form of drug abuse treatment and may be seen by patients as less stigmatizing than other treatment approaches. They are free of charge, widely available, and extremely valuable in offering support for sobriety and abstinence. Twelve-Step programs have a strong "recovery" orientation and a philosophy that emphasizes a medication-free approach to treatment. Although they are very helpful to those drug users who are motivated to make use of them, the Twelve-Step programs may have limited value for some injection drug users, and may not be a potent enough intervention to stop or significantly reduce needle use. An important future direction for self-help programs may be the development of specialized Twelve-Step groups for HIV-infected individuals.

Residential Treatment Programs

Residential drug abuse programs represent a second major treatment modality. These programs are rooted in the therapeutic community model, promulgated by such seminal programs as New York City's Daytop Village and Phoenix House, as well as San Francisco's Walden House and others. These programs offer a long-term residential setting, usually of 6 to 8 months' duration. Therapeutic communities can provide a powerful peer milieu that is designed to produce behavioral changes in the drug user (De Leon, 1984). Principles of treatment include the use of peer support, confrontation, and behavior shaping through the use of milieu-based rewards and punishments. Only a minority of drug users are motivated enough to voluntarily seek entry to these long-term and demanding programs; others enter as a result of legal coercion. Of those who do join, only a minority stay until completion. However, for those injection drug users who stay in treatment, residential therapeutic communities offer an effective tool for change. Residential programs have recently begun to address the special problems of treating HIV-infected clients (Galea, Lewis, & Baker, 1988; Goldstein & Yuen, 1988).

Although more residential treatment programs are beginning to accept HIV-infected injection drug users as clients, a number of thorny problems can complicate treatment. Motivating HIV-infected patients to seek admission to treatment can be difficult for any drug abuse treatment modality, and it is perhaps an even greater problem for residential programs because of their high demands. Traditionally, it has been necessary for drug users to demonstrate a high level of motivation and commitment as a prerequisite for acceptance into a long-term residential therapeutic community. Many HIV-infected drug users experience a sense of hopelessness (Batki et al., 1990c) and may lack the optimistic sense of an open-ended future that can be necessary in making long-term therapeutic commitments. Residential programs, therefore, need to increase their flexibility and lower their thresholds for admission of HIV-infected clients.

There are other problems facing residential programs as they attempt to work within the framework of the AIDS epidemic. These problems stem from the medical aspects of HIV disease. Residential therapeutic communities are usually not set up to provide the medical monitoring, evaluation, and treatment required by physically ill residents. Related problems involve the question of when to move a sick resident from the therapeutic community to a hospital or hospice. In general, a recurrent question is to what degree the needs of the community should be subordinate to the medical and psychological needs of an individual resident with AIDS or AIDS-related complex (ARC). For example, confrontation and behavioral limit setting may be difficult to enforce as strictly with sick patients as with healthy residents. This may lead to inconsistencies that can undermine the residential treatment milieu.

Medical Outpatient Treatments for Drug Abuse

Outpatient treatments generally belong to two main groups: "drug-free" treatments and medical treatments. Drug-free treatments employ individual or group psychotherapy combined with a variety of ancillary services such as vocational counseling. Since individual and group counseling approaches with HIV-infected injection drug users are covered in other chapters in this book, this section focuses on medical treatment, specifically MMT. Medically based treatments in outpatient drug abuse settings utilize pharmacological approaches that are specific for each class of drugs. For example, benzodiazepines are used for alcohol withdrawal; disulfiram for alcohol dependence; antidepressants and other agents for cocaine dependence; and clonidine, naltrexone, or methadone for the treatment of opiate dependence.

Most injection drug users in the United States are primary opiate users, whose drug of choice is generally heroin. Although nonmedical treatments such as self-help programs and residential therapeutic communities play important roles, by far the largest treatment modality for injection drug users follows a medical model—MMT. As many as 100,000 patients receive methadone treatment in the United States, in over 600 programs (U.S. General Accounting Office, 1990). Of these, about 80,000 patients are in MMT programs, while most of the rest are in 21-day methadone detoxification programs. A small number of patients receive methadone during inpatient hospitalization, and a few others are in longer detoxification programs lasting 21–180 days.

MMT provides a modality of last resort for patients who have failed at other treatments or for those who cannot or will not enter other forms of treatment. Long-term treatment with methadone is generally effective in greatly reducing injection opiate use and associated criminality (Ball et al., 1988; Senay, 1985). Short-term (21-day) treatment, such as methadone detoxification, is usually inadequate and inappropriate for HIV-infected patients. Detoxification is rarely successful in stopping injection drug use even in "healthy" injection drug users, and may have an even smaller chance of success among a more highly stressed group, such as patients with HIV infection. Long-term MMT does, however, offer a number of benefits for HIV-infected patients. MMT programs offer an ongoing, stable treatment setting within which medical, psychiatric, and social services can be offered in addition to substance abuse treatment (Batki, 1988).

Although methadone is the medical treatment of choice for opiate addiction, other medications are also effective. For example, clonidine is a useful nonaddictive agent to counteract acute opiate withdrawal symptoms (Gold, Redmond, & Kleber, 1978), but probably has a lesser role in the long-term treatment of HIV-infected injection drug users. Naltrexone, the long-acting oral opiate antagonist, can be very useful for those patients motivated enough to comply with such treatment (Kleber, 1985). Our experience at the SFGH Substance Abuse Services has been that very few HIV-infected opiate addicts are future-oriented, hopeful, or motivated enough to choose naltrexone treatment over long-term MMT. Buprenorphine is another agent that may be useful in opioid dependence. This is an investigational agent that may be effective as an alternative to methadone, and is discussed later in this chapter (Johnson, Cone, Henningfield, & Fudala, 1989).

A DRUG ABUSE TREATMENT PROGRAM FOR HIV-INFECTED INJECTION DRUG USERS

Mary: Early in Treatment

Mary has just completed her third month of MMT with mixed results to date. Although she has significantly cut back her heroin use from several times per day to about once per week, she still uses cocaine, alcohol, and sedative drugs fairly frequently, and has epileptic seizures related to her drug use. Members of the MMT program staff have confronted her regarding her "dirty" urine tests, but they are reluctant to threaten Mary with termination of treatment, because they are aware that she is HIV-infected and has a child to care for. Mary tells her counselor that she has trouble giving up drugs when she is not sure how long she has left to live. Her counselor understands that Mary is still in the early phase of treatment and is just beginning to cope with the trauma of having tested positive for HIV antibody.

Description of the Program

The staff of the SFGH Substance Abuse Services has developed and prospectively evaluated a specialized substance abuse treatment program, called the Program for AIDS Counseling and Education (PACE). PACE is aimed at injection drug users with AIDS, ARC, or asymptomatic HIV infection, and their sexual and drug-using partners (Sorensen, Batki, Good, & Wilkinson, 1989a). The program offers MMT, medical care, individual and group counseling, and AIDS prevention education. Patients attending the program are a heterogeneous group: Minorities are overrepresented, nearly 40% are women, 15% are homosexual or bisexual, and several families have children with AIDS. Patients are referred by AIDS treatment providers and by epidemiology research groups who test injection drug users for HIV infection. Preferential admission to methadone treatment services is given to HIV-infected patients.

PACE has adopted a policy of preferentially admitting HIV-infected injection drug users for three reasons. First, in San Francisco, the seroprevalence rate among injection drug users is well under 20%. This rate is relatively low when compared to many urban areas in the Northeast, where seroprevalence exceeds 50%. Because of the limited availability of drug abuse treatment resources in San Francisco, it was projected that these resources might have greater impact if focused on a specific group of injection drug users. Because the majority of San Francisco injection drug users are still seronegative, it was decided that a preferential admission policy should target the smaller group of seropositive injection drug users, in order to remove as many infectious individuals as possible from the pool of potential needle users and needle sharers. Second, preferential admission also facilitates educating and treating seropositive injection drug users. Third, preferentially admitting seropositive injection drug users addresses the need to slow the rate of disease progression among infected injection drug users. The SFGH MMT program provides on-site primary medical care and AIDS-related care to injection drug users. Tertiary prevention of HIV disease can be accomplished by providing zidovudine (AZT), aerosolized pentamidine, and other medical treatments in the setting of a drug abuse treatment program. This may be an important public health strategy, in that slowing the disease progression in infected injection drug users may reduce the cost of HIV disease to the individual and the community.

Methadone treatment of HIV-infected opiate users requires a number of changes from usual treatment approaches. Simply put, greater flexibility is needed in the care of these patients. HIV-infected patients generally present with far more psychosocial problems than other drug users do (Batki, Sorensen, Faltz, & Madover, 1988b). Psychological distress is high, especially in the form of depression and suicidality. More than one of every eight PACE patients entering treatment up to 1990 reported suicide attempts in the month prior to admission (Batki et al., 1990c). Distress of these proportions makes substance abuse treatment more difficult. HIV-infected patients may therefore need more time than other addicts to "clean up" their drug use. Another area needing greater flexibility is treatment duration. Methadone programs have traditionally encouraged their patients to try to taper off methadone and eventually live drug-free lives. Unfortunately, addicts can rarely stay drug-free for long, following discontinuation of methadone treatment. Since most addicts resume drug use after stopping methadone treatment, HIV-infected patients may find that the personal and public health costs of getting off methadone may be too high. Methadone-dosing strategies for HIV-infected patients also need to be flexible. Because of their high levels of psychological distress and physical discomfort, PACE patients are on average treated with higher methadone doses than are healthy patients. Conversely, for some patients (particularly those with impaired respiratory function or central nervous system disease), very low doses of methadone are indicated. Finally, somewhat more tolerance is needed for behavioral problems, although the line must be drawn at violent or threatening behavior. Because of both the personal health risks and the public health risks involved, great efforts are generally made to avoid treatment termination for HIV-infected patients. An alternative to termination is a temporary suspension from treatment, followed by readmission. The PACE clinic has employed temporary suspension rather than discharge from treatment as a form of limit setting for patients whose continued drug use would have led to discharge from traditional MMT. The experience of PACE is that some form of limit setting is required, even with HIV-infected patients, especially when all other treatment interventions have failed. Unfortunately, even some HIV-infected patients may eventually have to be discharged if their continuation in treatment is judged to be dangerous to patients or staff, or harmful to the treatment program as a whole.

Studies indicate that setting limits on drug-using behavior has a beneficial role in improving outcome in MMT (McCarthy & Borders, 1985; Calsyn & Saxon, 1987). At the SFGH MMT program, suspension from treatment consists of a 4- to 5-week taper from methadone, followed by a 30-day interruption of treatment. After the 30-day hiatus, a patient may be reconsidered for admission if willing to participate in additional adjunctive treatment modalities, such as a Twelve-Step self-help program, day treatment, residential treatment, or intensive counseling.

PACE distinguishes suspension from discharge, in that a patient who has been suspended from MMT is invited to apply for readmission into treatment. Suspension is a form of limit setting. It is frequently used as a "last-ditch" approach to informing patients that they are not complying with treatment expectations. Suspension also protects the integrity of the treatment milieu by enforcing behavioral standards for the clinic. Finally, suspension limits the possible contagion of high-risk behavior, such as drug use or sale, among patients.

Drug Abuse Treatment Outcome in This Program

Despite concerns that the increased severity of problems faced by these patients might reduce the effectiveness of MMT, the experience of the SFGH PACE has been promising. The first 42 HIV-infected patients who were prospectively evaluated in a treatment study showed significant decreases in several measures of drug use. Of the 21 subjects studied after 12 months of MMT, overall injection drug use decreased from an average of 27 days per month at entry into treatment to less than 6 days (see Figure 6.1). In particular, heroin use after 12 months of treatment decreased from 27 days to less than 4 days per month. Most of these significant decreases in injection drug use, and specifically heroin use, occurred after just 3 months of MMT (Batki, Sorensen, Coates, & Gibson, 1989).

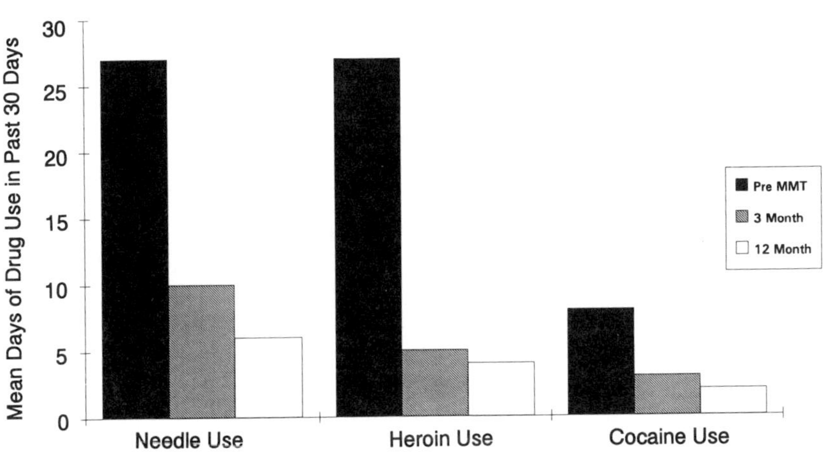

FIGURE 6.1. Needle, heroin, and cocaine use at 12 months among MMT patients in PACE (n = 21). Adapted from S. L. Batki, J. L. Sorensen, D. R. Gibson, and P. Maude-Griffin (1990c).

Even though methadone treatment is not a specific therapy for stimulant abuse, the same study showed that cocaine use also decreased after 3 months of treatment, from an average of 8 days to less than 3 days per month. Outcome, however, is heavily influenced by psychiatric factors and is discussed below.

Stimulant Abuse Treatment for This Population

The treatment of stimulant abuse may be particularly important in the prevention of AIDS. Because of its short duration of effect, cocaine users must readminister the drug frequently, increasing their exposure to potentially contaminated needles. As Chapter 3 has explained, cocaine use has been implicated as an especially important risk factor for HIV infection for injection drug users (Chaisson et al., 1989). There is no single currently accepted medical treatment for cocaine abuse. Although a number of medications have been proposed or tried in recent years, none of them have achieved the widespread application of methadone treatment for opiate addiction. Some new treatments for stimulant abuse employ pharmacotherapy in the form of tricyclic antidepressants, particularly desipramine. Some antidepressant studies have been promising (Gawin, 1988), but others have failed to replicate the utility of desipramine for cocaine abuse, particularly in MMT patients (Arndt, Dorozynsky, Woody, McLellan, & O'Brien, 1988). Other investigators have looked to dopamine agonists, such as the antiparkinsonian drugs amantadine and bromocriptine, to decrease the postabstinence craving for cocaine (Tennant & Sagherian, 1987; Dackis, Gold, Davies, & Sweeney, 19851986). To date, however, both antidepressants and antiparkinsonian drugs are useful, but there is no firm evidence to support the uniform application of one treatment over the other. Furthermore, although medications are important adjuncts, psychosocial interventions remain crucial to cocaine abuse treatment.

Cocaine use is a prominent problem in MMT populations (Chambers, Taylor, & Moffett, 1972; Kaul & Davidow, 1981; Kosten, Morgan, & Kleber, 1990; Kosten, Rounsaville, & Kleber, 1987; Strug, Hunt, Goldsmith, Lipton, & Spunt, 1985). Some studies have indicated that cocaine use may increase when drug users undergo MMT (Chaisson et al., 1989). In an attempt to reduce cocaine abuse among MMT patients, Kosten et al. (1990) employed a trial of buprenorphine, a mixed opioid agonistantagonist, which has been used investigatively in treating opioid dependence. Buprenorphine may be particularly useful with MMT patients who also abuse cocaine. MMT patients treated with buprenorphine, rather than methadone, demonstrated significantly less cocaine use (Kosten et al., 1989). Kosten and colleagues speculated that buprenorphine, as a partial agonist, may have less of a "speedball" effect when combined with cocaine than does methadone. In addition, the partial agonist properties of buprenorphine may diminish the attractiveness of heroin–cocaine combinations by partially blocking the effects of the heroin portion of the combination.

In response to the increase in cocaine abuse among MMT at SFGH—especially those with HIV infection—two treatment studies were recently conducted at SFGH to determine the effectiveness of group therapy and with and without added pharmacotherapy in decreasing cocaine abuse. In the first of these studies (Batki, Manfredi, & Dumontet, 1990b), the impact of a 12-week course of psychoeducational group therapy was examined. Weekly group therapy, employing a model that combined psychoeducation, supportive counseling, and relapse prevention training, was used in an attempt to reduce cocaine abuse. The treatment response of these patients was prospectively evaluated. Ten of the 13 participating patients were HIV-infected, and the majority used cocaine intravenously. Treatment outcome was disappointing, even though group attendance was surprisingly good (all but two of the patients attended at least 10 of the 12 scheduled sessions). Patients reported an increased sense of control over their cocaine use; unfortunately, however, no significant changes occurred in cocaine use when assessed either by patient self-report or objective measures such as urine testing.

A second study (Batki et al., 1991) examined the treatment of 16 cocaine-dependent MMT patients with a 9-week combination of fluoxetine and weekly psychoeducational group therapy. Eleven out of the 16 patients were HIV-infected, and 10 had a lifetime history of Major Depressive Disorder. The antidepressant fluoxetine was administered each morning in an open outpatient 9-week trial, with doses ranging from 20 to 60 mg per day. The average final doses for fluoxetine and methadone were, respectively, 45 mg and 52 mg per day. By the ninth week, patients reported significant decreases in their cocaine use, cocaine craving, and money spent buying cocaine. Patient reports were supplemented by the analysis of urine cocaine and benzoylecgonine levels, and these measures supported that patients were indeed significantly decreasing their cocaine use. Group therapy may therefore be necessary, but not sufficient, to successfully treat HIV-infected cocaine dependent patients in MMT. These patients may need to be treated with a combination of pharmacotherapy and group therapy. Further research is needed to determine how existing psychotherapeutic strategies for opiate-dependent patients can be modified to fit the special needs of the HIV-infected cocaine abuser in outpatient MMT.

Ancillary Services Provided through Drug Abuse Treatment

In addition to methadone treatment, outpatient drug treatment programs need to provide medical, psychiatric, and social services for HIV-infected injection drug users. Drug abuse treatment programs traditionally have only had the resources to provide the bare minimum of such services. This minimum is no longer enough when drug abuse treatment programs face a severely ill and increasingly disabled population. Injection drug users have a difficult time making and keeping the numerous appointments with various health care and social service providers involved in their treatment. This means that drug programs must do more to establish liaisons with other treatment providers, and may need to provide ancillary services at the treatment site. Examples are the on-site provision of psychiatric evaluation and treatment and AIDS-related medical care at drug programs. Such services, by providing better day-to-day care for HIV-infected injection drug users, may reduce the number and severity of psychiatric and medical crises that might otherwise lead to more intense and expensive interventions, such as hospitalization.

MEDICAL TREATMENT

Mary: Integrated AIDS Medical Services

After 5 months of treatment in MMT, Mary is still relatively asymptomatic from her HIV disease. Although she has few somatic symptoms other than fatigue and night sweats, she has experienced psychological symptoms of depression associated with her awareness of worrisome laboratory test abnormalities, such as a progressive T (helper) lymphocyte depletion. Mary has been followed medically since entry into MMT. The program physician and nurse practitioner have periodically tested and examined her, in consultation with the SFGH AIDS clinic physician, who is present at the drug program on a weekly basis. Mary has been started on AZT in order to slow the progression of HIV disease. Because Mary's life is still turbulent and unstable, being able to get her medical treatment at the MMT program makes it easier for her to comply with medical care.

HIV-infected MMT patients often have substantial medical problems (Brown, Chu, Nemoto, Ajuluchkwu, & Primm, 1989), but a full spectrum of primary medical care is infrequently provided at outpatient methadone programs (Selwyn et al., 1989). Drug users are often unreliable in seeking medical care in traditional health care settings. Health care professionals at several AIDS clinics are wary of treating substance abusers, because they perceive these patients as noncompliant with treatment (Samuels, 1990). Thus, many HIV-infected injection drug users in outpatient drug treatment may not be receiving timely medical care that could slow the progression of their HIV disease. Developing primary medical care services for HIV-infected injection drug users could relieve the morbidity and fiscal costs associated with HIV disease.

The outpatient MMT clinic at SFGH has been treating increasing numbers of HIV-infected injection drug users. Because of the preferential admissions policy for HIV-infected patients, by August 1990 approximately 110 out of 190 patients in the MMT clinic were HIV-infected. To meet their health care needs, the SFGH Substance Abuse Services staff has developed a program for on-site primary HIV-related medical care delivery for MMT patients. Patients receive early monitoring for HIV infection, and infected patients are treated with medications such as AZT and aerosolized pentamidine. Services are provided by the MMT medical staff, with assistance from the SFGH AIDS clinic. A recent study (Batki et al., 1990a) of the new on-site primary medical care clinic revealed that medical services are heavily used by HIV-infected injection drug users in MMT. Medical visits at the SFGH MMT clinic were compared before and after the addition of AIDS primary care and the availability of weekly AIDS clinic specialty consultation to the MMT program. After the addition of these enriched AIDS medical services, there was a significant increase in medical visits. Analysis of medical visits made to the MMT clinic in 1989 showed that most of the medical visits were made by the HIV-infected injection drug users, who utilized medical care out of proportion to their actual numbers in the clinic. HIV-infected patients, although constituting less than 50% of the total clinic population at the time of the study, made over 80% of the medical visits at the program (see Figure 6.2). Of the medical contacts made by HIV-infected injection drug users, the majority were for the treatment of somatic symptoms, as compared to the substance-abuse-related and psychiatric complaints that accounted for the majority of medical contacts for non-HIV-infected MMT patients.

This study demonstrated that HIV-infected injection drug users require a far greater proportion of medical services than seronegative injection drug users. In addition, HIV-infected injection drug users are more likely than other MMT patients to require treatment for medical symptoms than for psychiatric or substance abuse problems. Another important finding in this study was that over half of the medical contacts with HIV-infected patients were made on a "drop-in" basis rather than by appointment. This points to the importance of the flexibility that can be provided by on-site care available on a daily basis. Injection

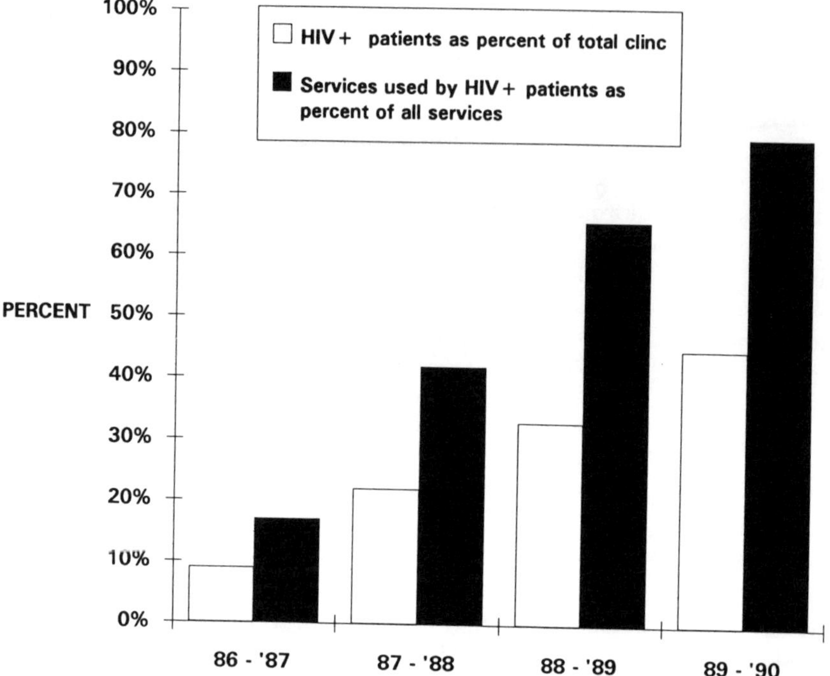

FIGURE 6.2. Medical services utilized by HIV-positive injection drug users. Adapted from S. L. Batki, J. London, E. Goosby, M. Clement, R. Wolfe, C. Ryan, D. French, M. Young, D. Miller, R. Christmas, and J. Sorensen (1990a, June).

drug users in MMT are responsive to such on-site medical care. Medical services for AIDS and ARC can therefore be provided effectively in a methadone treatment program, with some assistance and consultation from an AIDS clinic.

PSYCHIATRIC ASPECTS OF TREATMENT

Mary: Psychiatric Problems

Mary's continued drug use, marital turmoil, and inability to care for her child have led to the child's removal from her home, following a report made to the child protective services by Mary's MMT counselor. The loss of her child and the impact of HIV disease have led to a worsening of Mary's depression and drug use. She has voiced suicidal thoughts, necessitating almost daily contact with the program psychiatrist for evaluation of suicidal potential. It becomes clear that outpatient MMT is no longer adequate for Mary. A treatment plan is created, referring Mary to drug abuse day treatment and psychiatric residential care in addition to remaining in MMT, where she will continue to receive methadone treatment, counseling, and medical care for HIV disease.

There are several major areas of mental health service needs related to AIDS and drug abuse. These include educational counseling to prevent AIDS, drug abuse treatment, and mental health treatment of HIV-infected drug users (including consultation with medical treatment providers). These needs are difficult to meet, not only because of a scarcity of resources, but because of the complexity of the interactions among the different systems that are required to coordinate the care of patients with drug abuse, mental health, and medical problems.

Counseling specific to AIDS must be part of treatment programs for intravenous drug users. A basic component of such counseling is education concerning safe sex and the importance of avoiding the sharing of needles. Counseling departs from usual substance abuse treatment in a number of ways. Family and couples counseling may be necessary to help patients and their families come to terms with the changes associated with HIV disease. Grief counseling is needed to help patients to cope with the deaths of friends or spouses, and with the fear of their own illness or death. Patients also need the opportunity to deal with feelings of grief about other sorts of losses, such as the inability to work or loss of sexuality (Batki, 1988). Individual counseling aimed at these difficult issues can be supplemented by referral of patients to support groups designed to meet some of the special needs of HIV-infected patients.

Types of Psychiatric Problems in This Population

Drug abuse treatment of HIV-infected patients faces difficulties resulting from the severity of the multiple problems presented by its target population. It is particularly difficult to motivate HIV-infected patients, who may suffer from anxiety, depression, or demoralization, possibly combined with physical discomfort. Appeals both to altruism and to self-interest are two counseling strategies that may help to motivate HIV-infected patients. Counselors can attempt to evoke a sense of altruism through educational counseling that aims to teach injection drug users that using needles and sharing needles can spread HIV from the patient to others whom the addict cares about, such as friends and family. This message is essentially "Don't use drugs, because you may spread AIDS to others." The second approach—appeal to self-interest or preservation of health—can also be presented in didactic counseling.

This approach addresses the likelihood of increased morbidity associated with continued needle use, based on the probability that continued parenteral exposure to foreign antigens may be an activating cofactor for HIV (Zagury et al., 1986), and on some tentative evidence that decreased needle use may be associated with decreased morbidity in infected injection drug users (Des Jarlais et al., 1987b).

Even without the impact of AIDS, psychiatric problems are common among drug users. The majority of drug users have other diagnosable psychiatric disorders (Rounsaville, Weissman, Kleber, & Wilber, 1982b). When AIDS, ARC, or asymptomatic HIV infection is added to drug abuse, the risks for psychopathology increase. There are a number of common sources of psychological distress among drug users with HIV disease. Although these stressors tend to be similar to those faced by non-drug-using HIV patients, they are made more severe by the special vulnerabilities of drug users. Some of these sources of distress include awareness of one's terminal illness; losses of health and sexuality; isolation and ostracism; and the negative attitudes or countertransference of health care providers. Psychiatric problems are particularly important, in that they can exacerbate drug use. The poor coping skills and common ego deficits noted in these patients (Khantzian, Mack, & Schatzberg, 1974; Khantzian, 1979) may lead them to respond to the added stresses of illness by increasing their drug use. Drug users may not have other adaptive mechanisms that are effective enough to control the dysphoria that can result from stress. In fact, mood disorders and anxiety disorders are among the most common psychiatric disorders seen in drug users (Rounsaville, Weissman, Crits-Cristoph, Wilber, & Kleber, 1982a).

Pre-existing psychopathology is only one of the multiple contributions to the mental health problems of HIV-infected drug users. A second contributing factor is continued drug use, with its associated acute and chronic psychiatric sequelae. A third source of psychiatric problems is HIV itself—its direct effects on the brain, such as HIV encephalopathy (AIDS dementia), and its indirect effects, such as secondary infections or neoplasms involving the central nervous system. Finally, the psychosocial factors associated with AIDS, such as isolation, ostracism, and the impact of losses, make up yet another layer of additive stress that contributes to mental health problems. The psychological themes voiced by these patients include denial, anger and antisocial behavior, depression, isolation, and continued drug abuse (Batki et al., 1988).

Psychiatric disorders have been encountered in the majority of the HIV-infected drug users in treatment at SFGH. For example, in a sample of 49 HIV-infected injection drug users in MMT referred for psychiatric consultation, 84% had a Diagnostic and Statistical Manual of

Mental Disorders, third edition, revised (DSM-III-R) psychiatric diagnosis. Thirty-three percent had depressive disorders, another 33% had anxiety disorders, and 18% had organic brain syndromes.

Psychiatric disorders among drug users are especially important, in that they are associated with worse treatment outcome, and (by extension) possibly greater risks of spreading HIV. Psychiatric severity in drug users has been shown to be a predictor of poor outcome in drug abuse treatment (McLellan, Luborsky, & Woody, 1983). Research at SFGH strongly suggests that this relationship also holds true for HIV-infected injection drug users (Batki et al., 1990b). In a prospective study of drug abuse treatment outcome, depression, hopelessness, and suicidality at intake into treatment of HIV-infected patients were predictive of worse outcome in terms of heroin, cocaine, and total injection drug use 1 year later (see Figure 6.3). At the start of MMT, 60% of these subjects had moderate to high levels of depression on the Beck Depression Inventory (Beck, Ward, Mendelson, Mock, & Erbaugh, 1961), and the majority also had moderate or higher levels of hopelessness as measured by the Beck Hopelessness Scale (Beck, Weissman, Lester, & Trexler, 1975). Almost three-quarters of these HIV-infected patients complained of depression in the month prior to entry, and 37% reported having thoughts of suicide, with as many as 13% of subjects reporting that they had made a suicide attempt in the month prior to entry. Those patients who reported initial depression had six times

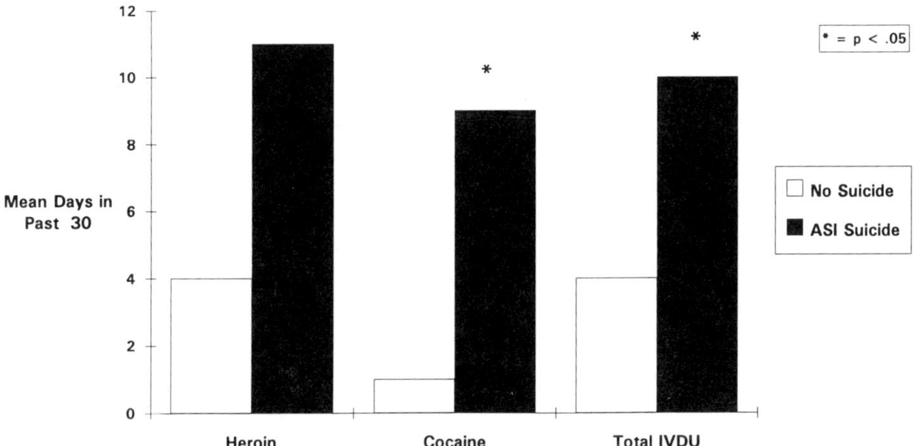

FIGURE 6.3. ASI suicidality at intake as a predicator of 12-month drug abuse outcome among HIV-infected patients (intake n = 42). Adapted from S. L. Batki, J. L. Sorenson, D. R. Gibson, and P. Maude-Griffin (1990c).

as many days of injection drug use at 12 months of treatment as subjects who denied depression. Subjects with reports of suicidality at intake also reported many more days of drug use (especially cocaine) at 12 months of treatment, as compared to patients without suicidality. The prevalence and prognostic significance of psychological distress among these patients point to the need for early identification and intervention for psychiatric problems.

Levels of Mental Health Care

Managing the psychiatric problems seen in HIV-infected drug users requires at least six different levels of multidisciplinary interventions involving drug abuse counselors, social workers, psychotherapists, and physicians. Perhaps the most important level of intervention is the provision of concrete forms of practical, material assistance and support. The diagnosis of HIV seropositivity, ARC, or AIDS is often accompanied by distress. Patients may experience anxiety associated with the sense of uncertainty they experience about their disease: its severity, its time course, its treatments. Anything that can be done to reduce this uncertainty may be of help to patients. Material supports such as assistance with housing, welfare funds, meals, transportation, and health care serve to reduce uncertainty and accompanying anxiety.

A second type of intervention consists of providing patients with helpful information. Education can have a powerful effect in reducing uncertainty and helplessness. Self-help groups are a third level of intervention and are important in reducing isolation. These groups, however, may be difficult to provide for drug users, who may lack a supportive community or peers willing and able to provide a self-help treatment milieu. Supportive psychotherapy is a fourth level of mental health intervention. The goal of such therapy is to support defenses rather than to uncover or analyze them, because drug users may suffer from poorly developed defensive ego mechanisms even before the onset of HIV disease. Supportive psychotherapy, however, must still confront the self-destructive behaviors that many injection drug users may continue to engage in even after infection with HIV.

A fifth level of mental health intervention may be the use of psychiatric medications if psychotherapy alone is inadequate. This is particularly necessary in the presence of serious mood and anxiety disorders, psychosis, and "organic" disorders such as dementia. The cornerstone of pharmacological management of HIV-infected injection drug users is safety. Treatment should not be allowed to increase morbidity by adding medication-related adverse effects to the effects of AIDS and drug abuse. Drug abusers may not be able to safely handle potentially abusable medications such as benzodiazepines and psychostimulants. An example of a nonaddictive, relatively safe psychiatric medication is buspirone, which may have some utility as an alternative to the benzodiazepines in the treatment of chronic anxiety in HIV-infected drug users. We have reported the results of treating a group of 17 HIV-infected MMT patients with buspirone (Batki, 1990). All of these patients showed at least temporary improvement in one or more of the following areas: subjective reduction of anxiety; reduction of prescribed benzodiazepine use; or reduction in positive urine tests for drugs of abuse, particularly morphine. Buspirone was well tolerated in all but three of these patients, and there was no evidence of buspirone misuse. Given its benign adverse effect profile, buspirone may be particularly useful in the treatment of anxiety in HIV-infected drug users.

If outpatient strategies fail, residential treatment may be required. Such treatment can take the form of halfway houses or other alternatives to hospitalization. However, hospitalization may be needed when it becomes necessary to protect patients from hurting themselves or others, or to support the patient who cannot provide for basic self-care needs. Throughout this entire sequence of levels of intervention, the mental health provider must negotiate the complex problems of dealing not merely with a "dual diagnosis," but with a "triple diagnosis": drug abuse and psychiatric problems in the presence of HIV disease. Mental health interventions may need to follow a case management model, because patients will require frequent contacts, extensive networking with different agencies, and negotiation with a variety of service providers. Often, it is difficult to find treatment settings that can handle the concurrent presentation of psychiatric disorder, drug abuse, related antisocial behaviors, and medical problems. Managing these triple-diagnosis patients is a growing challenge for the field of mental health. Further work is urgently needed to develop effective models of treatment for HIV-infected drug users.

AIDS PREVENTION WITH ETHNIC AND SEXUAL MINORITIES

Ethnic and sexual minority injection drug users are at particularly high risk for HIV infection (Brown & Primm, 1989; Peterson & Bakeman, 1989; Peterson & Marin, 1988). AIDS prevention campaigns in drug treatment clinics would be incomplete without addressing how best to serve these groups. Substance abuse treatment programs, such as those utilizing MMT, may face difficulties in reaching ethnic and sexual minority injection drug users. This section describes some of these difficulties, and points to directions for future work to improve AIDS prevention services for these patients.

Ethnic minority injection drug users have been described as having special treatment and AIDS prevention needs (Brown & Primm, 1989; Marin & Marin, 1990; Bean, 1989; Crespo, 1989). Some African-American injection drug users, for example, may perceive AIDS as being a disease of gay men and may associate AIDS with loss of masculinity (Stall & Ostrow, 1989). Injection drug users who deny homosexual risk behaviors for HIV infection may be less knowledgeable about HIV transmission through sexual relations (Stall & Ostrow, 1989). These clients may therefore need focused education regarding the sexual transmission of AIDS. Another potential focus for AIDS prevention and education for minority injection drug users in treatment programs is condom use. African-American and Hispanic women may have special needs for support and education regarding safe sex (M. T. Fullilove, Fullilove, Haynes, & Gross, 1990a; Wermuth, Ham, & Robbins, 1991). Research has shown that psychoeducational approaches to AIDS prevention can be effective when aimed specifically at African-American and Hispanic people who are at high risk for AIDS (M. T. Fullilove, Fullilove, & Morales, 1989).

Sexual minorities may present different prevention and clinical challenges than injection drug users from ethnic minority communities. As a group, gay, lesbian, and bisexual injection drug users have received less attention in drug treatment. Gays, lesbians, bisexuals, and injection drug users with sexual identity problems may also have different AIDS prevention and treatment needs than heterosexual injection drug users. These differences may be difficult for drug treatment programs to address. One approach is to refer homosexual injection drug users to community agencies that are identified as serving homosexuals. Unfortunately, these referrals may not always be successful, since gay injection drug users are not very well connected to the homosexual community at large (Stall & Ostrow, 1989).

Several AIDS prevention campaigns have been successfully implemented with drug-free gay men (McKusick, Conant, & Coates, 1985a; Kelly, St. Lawrence, Hood, & Brasfield, 1989). However, these interventions still await to be implemented with gay male injection drug users in treatment. Drug abuse treatment clinicians may need to receive training to meet the AIDS prevention and treatment needs of gay and lesbian clients. Future AIDS prevention programs situated in drug treatment sites may better serve ethnic and sexual minority injection drug users by providing interventions that are culturally specific and are inclusive of injection drug users of all sexual orientations.

FUTURE DIRECTIONS FOR RESEARCH AND TREATMENT

Drug abuse treatment settings are effective sites for AIDS prevention with injection drug users (Batki et al., 1990a; Selwyn et al., 1989). Clinical interventions with HIV-infected injection drug users in outpatient drug abuse treatment, specifically in MMT programs, are apparently helpful in reducing drug use and therefore potentially controlling the spread of AIDS (Batki et al., 1989; Serraino & Franceschi, 1990; Williams et al., 1990). The provision of on-site primary medical care to opiate addicts in MMT clinics is an important innovation in drug treatment with injection drug users, particularly those already HIV-infected (Batki et al., 1990a; Samuels, 1990). These approaches may help slow the progression of illness in those already infected. Psychotropic medications such as fluoxetine and buspirone may be helpful psychopharmacological interventions for HIV-infected injection drug users with psychiatric and polydrug (e.g., opiate plus cocaine) problems. HIV-infected injection drug users may be particularly helped by drug treatment programs that have modified their definition of recovery and expectations about treatment outcome, and that can incorporate AIDS prevention objectives into treatment planning. The greater availability of ancillary services, such as social services, grief counseling, and liaison with other agencies, has also benefited seropositive injection drug users.

Although outpatient drug treatment programs are beginning to meet the special needs of HIV-infected patients, programs are still early in the process of exploring interventions specifically tailored for those HIV-infected injection drug users addicted to cocaine. Psychopharmacological agents may be useful for this group of addicts, particularly if they are used to supplement group psychotherapy. Seropositive injection drug users in drug treatment benefit from a variety of clinical interventions that are well integrated into drug abuse treatment planning and are responsive to their multiple needs. Multidisciplinary approaches to outpatient drug treatment appear to be the best defense against the spread of AIDS.

Self-help and residential programs have important roles in reducing drug abuse and preventing AIDS, but may be limited in their abilities to treat HIV-infected patients with serious medical and psychiatric problems. These treatment modalities seem to have their greatest strength in helping seronegative injection drug users pursue more traditional approaches to recovery from substance abuse. Research is needed to examine how to make self-help groups and therapeutic communities more accessible and appropriate for seropositive addicts, who may be limited in their ability to utilize these programs in their current forms.

Although outpatient MMT programs in the United States are increasingly successful in providing comprehensive drug abuse, psychiatric, and medical care to HIV-infected injection drug users, some clinics, particularly in Europe and Australia, may be offering an even wider range of services (Donoghoe, Dolan, & Stimson, 1990; Lowe et al., 1990; Stimson & Lart, 1990). Future efforts may need to be devoted to exploring ways of amplifying clinical services, such as needle exchange, family planning, child care, dental care, and other services for underserved seropositive injection drug users. Finally, more research is needed to develop better psychotherapeutic and pharmacological treatment techniques for the HIV-infected injection drug user who abuses cocaine.

In summary, drug abuse treatment is an effective AIDS prevention strategy. Treatment programs are ideal sites for providing the integrated system of services needed by drug users, especially when they are already infected with HIV.

Chapter 7

Group Counseling to Prevent AIDS

JAMES L. SORENSEN
JULIE LONDON
EDUARDO S. MORALES

What can a staff member in a drug treatment program do to help prevent AIDS? As the AIDS epidemic advances, this question is facing counselors in drug abuse treatment programs ever more frequently. As Chapter 6 has noted, providing effective drug treatment is one important way to prevent the spread of AIDS, because drug abuse treatment can have direct effects on restricting the spread of HIV infection by decreasing injection drug use. Treatment can also have indirect effects by reaching drug users with information about AIDS and helping them to change the behaviors that put them at risk of acquiring or transmitting HIV. These educational effects may be more powerful, because they can last beyond the time of drug treatment, and they have the possibility of reaching beyond clients in programs—out to their fellow drug users who are not in treatment, their families, and their sexual partners. Also, treatment programs can foster social support for changing group norms regarding safety in needle use and sexual practices. But educational programs will be more effective if they are guided by theoretical and practical models. Chapter 5 has discussed how theoretical models can guide AIDS prevention programs for drug users. This chapter provides a practical model: the group approach.

Group interventions have been tested in several controlled AIDS prevention studies in drug treatment programs. In this chapter, we first explain the nature of this approach and then review the studies that have evaluated its effects. A second section reviews what is known about impact. A third section of the chapter is more practical: It presents detailed information about how to conduct such groups in a drug treatment program, drawing from our experience in conducting such groups in detoxification, methadone maintenance, and therapeutic community programs. In addition, AIDS prevention strategies with ethnic and sexual minority drug abusers are reviewed. The chapter concludes with suggestions about the areas where these groups seem most and least effective, finishing with suggestions for further development of this promising approach to preventing HIV infection.

WHAT ARE GROUP COUNSELING APPROACHES?

Group counseling approaches have seen anywhere from 4 to 50 drug treatment clients simultaneously, providing an intervention that encourages them to change the behaviors that spread HIV infection. Group counseling to prevent AIDS is a natural development for drug treatment programs. Group therapy is a potent intervention (Yalom, 1985), and it is a common treatment approach in drug programs (Lawson, 1984); thus, the group format fits well with the tradition of drug abuse treatment. The group format is also efficient, in that a small number of staff members can work with many clients. In addition, the group setting can build social support for change. For example, clients can enact scenarios that depict a drug user being offered a previously used (but drug-filled) syringe and discuss how to resist the social pressures to share needles.

The group approach also has limitations. The overwhelming needs or interactive style of some participants may mean that others get less attention. It can also be difficult to tailor the group format to the problems of every participant. For example, a man who recently received seropositive HIV test results has different psychological and educational needs than a woman who knows that she is seronegative and is thinking of becoming pregnant. Finally, intimate activities are linked to HIV transmission, and it can be difficult to discuss these in a group.

Group approaches have employed several of the conceptual premises discussed in the chapter on theory. The approach our group uses at the University of California, San Francisco (UCSF) is grounded in health psychology principles and literature on the health belief model (Beck & Frankel, 1981; Rogers, 1975; Rosenstock, 1974; see Chapter 5). Rather than using fear appeals alone, we try to portray AIDS as a real but controllable threat. Then in group sessions we try to increase participants' belief in the effectiveness of health care guidelines ("response efficacy"), to increase their belief that they can do the actions that will prevent HIV infection ("self-efficacy"), and to help them to develop the communication skills to resist pressures to engage in risky behaviors. In New York, Schilling, El-Bassel, Schinke, Gordon, and Nichols (1991) developed their skills-building program for female drug users around the same health belief model. Other researchers have employed other conceptual bases. For example, Magura et al. (in press) built their peer support groups on the models of brief psychotherapy (Haley, 1978; Blizinsky & Reid, 1980).

HOW EFFECTIVE ARE GROUPS?

Although this approach is experimental, several researchers have been evaluating the effectiveness of group interventions to slow the spread of HIV. We are aware of several investigators who have presented the results of controlled studies.

Outpatients

Working with drug abusers in outpatient programs, several researchers have demonstrated some evidence of efficacy to this approach. Magura and colleagues worked with 284 drug abusers in methadone maintenance programs (Magura et al., in press; Magura, Shapiro, Grossman, & Lipton, 1989; Magura, 1989). They matched clinics, then compared three interventions: (1) group education with a follow-up peer support group and HIV testing; (2) group education with follow-up peer support group (without antibody testing); and (3) no intervention. They found that those who went through the education learned more about their risk of HIV infection, and those who participated in the peer groups developed a more positive attitude toward condoms and reported more condom use. At Columbia University's program, Robert Schilling and colleagues worked with women on methadone maintenance (Schilling, El-Bassel, Gordon, & Nichols, 1989a; Schilling et al., in press). They randomly assigned 83 women drug abusers to receive a five-session skills-building group or to receive one session of standard information about AIDS. At a posttest, they found that the women who participated in the skills-building groups stated that they intended to have less sex with drug users; they were more likely to discuss safe sex with sexual partners; and they were more likely than those in the information condition to be carrying condoms.

Our work with drug abusers in outpatient programs in San Francisco has also yielded encouraging results (Heitzmann et al., 1989; Sorensen et al., 1989c; Sorensen, Gibson, Heitzmann, Dumontet, & Morales, 1989e; Sorensen, Heitzmann, & Guydish, 1990). With 50 methadone maintenance clients, we conducted a random assignment study in which half received a 6-hour AIDS prevention workshop and the other half received informational brochures. When workshop subjects were compared to controls after the intervention, workshop subjects showed superiority in these areas: factual knowledge about AIDS, knowledge about risk reduction practices in terms of sex, perceived drug-related self-efficacy, and ability to demonstrate the correct procedure for using a condom. When outcome was measured again at the 3-month follow-up, workshop subjects maintained their gains in these areas. Although controls and workshop subjects did not differ at the posttest in perceived self-efficacy in terms of sex and ability to demonstrate the correct procedure for needle sterilization, differences emerged at the 3-month follow-up, with workshop participants surpassing controls in both the needle sterilization demonstration and sex-related self-efficacy.

Ninety-eight subjects from the 21-day outpatient detoxification clinic at San Francisco General Hospital also participated in the study. Forty-nine of these were assigned to the 6-hour intervention, and the remaining 49 received a packet of educational brochures only. Regarding outcome measurement, there were clear differences at the postintervention interview. In comparison to controls, workshop subjects showed superior factual knowledge about AIDS, superior knowledge about risk reduction in terms of sexual behaviors, more anxiety about AIDS, and greater skill at demonstrating the correct procedure for using a condom. Some of these beneficial effects endured to a 3-month follow-up, including group differences in knowledge about AIDS risk reduction practices in terms of sex, anxiety about AIDS, and skill in demonstrating the correct procedure for using a condom. Differences in factual knowledge about AIDS and anxiety about AIDS between controls and workshop participants seemed to fade by the 3-month follow-up.

A study of 90-minute small-group counseling yielded negative results (Calsyn, Saxon, & Freeman, 1990). In this study, outpatient drug abusers, 75% of whom were in methadone maintenance, participated in a study that involved random assignment to a 90-minute group; to a group plus opportunity for HIV testing; or to a control condition that received the group after 4 months. The 313 subjects were followed up 4 months after the pretest. Most subjects in all three groups had lowered their HIV risk in the interim, and there were no significant effects of the experimental manipulations. Calsyn and colleagues' experience suggests that brief informational groups like this may be insufficient to produce measurable changes in clients' HIV risk.

Inpatients

Three research groups have reported the results of controlled studies of the efficacy of group education with drug abusers in residential care.

John Weber and colleagues worked with 100 drug abusers in a New York inpatient detoxification clinic, who were randomly assigned to two conditions: (1) small-group discussion sessions or (2) large-group discussions with videotapes and lectures (Weber, Dengelegi, Torquato, Kolakathis, & Yancovitz, 1989). Participants in both conditions improved their knowledge about AIDS, beliefs about risk, and intent to lower risky behaviors from a pre- to a postintervention assessment, and the two educational conditions did not differ in outcomes.

Our research team conducted a random assignment study with 96 residents of a drug-free therapeutic community, comparing a 6-hour group intervention with a brochures-only comparison condition (Sorensen, Gibson, Heitzmann, Dumontet, & Acampora, 1988b; Sorensen et al., 1989c, 1989d). There was a significant effect at the postintervention interview in knowledge of AIDS risk, and a statistical trend in the expected direction in self-efficacy. By 6 months the knowledge difference had deteriorated, but the differences in clients' perceived self-efficacy in avoiding HIV infection had become statistically significant.

A third study was carried out with residents in an inpatient detoxification facility, but its preliminary results are not encouraging (McCusker et al., 1990). These investigators found improvements in residents' attitudes and decreases in their HIV risk, but no differences between those who received 2 hours of information versus a 6-hour enhanced intervention.

To summarize, several researchers have evaluated group counseling approaches, working in outpatient and inpatient settings, using different methods and measures. In general, these have been tightly controlled experiments, and their varied results seem to show that small groups can affect patients' knowledge of AIDS and their attitudes toward HIV risk. However, the studies have not for the most part had a large influence on the participants' behavior. The behavioral changes observed, such as being more likely to carry condoms, are small. Generally, these studies show that the group approaches have promise.

HOW GROUPS WORK

At UCSF, our research team has developed psychoeducational AIDS prevention groups for injection drug users enrolled in a residential drug treatment program, an outpatient methadone maintenance clinic, and a 21-day outpatient detoxification clinic. These group interventions are intended (1) to increase the drug treatment clients' understanding of AIDS transmission and prevention; (2) to build skills that can help injection drug users avoid getting or spreading AIDS; and (3) to assist clients in making the necessary changes in lifestyle to protect themselves and others from contracting HIV. The AIDS prevention groups are designed for 4 to 10 clients, with two to three leaders.

Below we explain in some detail how these groups work, to give readers a sense of how we have translated the concepts of AIDS prevention into action. There is not enough information here for someone actually to run an effective group. For that, one can consult our training manual (Heitzmann et al., 1989). There is enough information, however, for personnel in treatment programs to determine whether or not such an approach would be feasible in their clinics, and to begin planning how they would tailor the group approach to their clientele.

Elements

This psychoeducational intervention combines elements of a semistructured, process-oriented group with a structured educational workshop. We conceptualize the counseling group in terms of five components:

1. *Didactic presentations* provide basic facts about AIDS transmission and prevention and define technical terms for group members. For example, the leaders describe the course of illness—from becoming infected, to developing symptomatic HIV disease, to an AIDS diagnosis.
2. *Group discussions* bring information "home" for group participants. They help personalize the threat of AIDS. For example, participants watch a videotape clip of injection drug users with AIDS discussing denial. Then the leaders ask how participants have seen denial of AIDS risks in their friends.
3. *Structured exercises* and homework give participants specific things to do, to build skills and decrease anxiety. For example, participants practice the correct ways to put on a condom, using materials provided in the workshop; they then take materials home with the assignment to teach someone else.
4. *Social interactions* build cohesion among group members and leaders, helping to build trust. For example, group participants pair up in the skill-building exercises; each partner rates and helps the other to learn the correct procedures for needle cleaning and condom use. In addition, the group shares refreshments during meetings, getting to know each other informally.
5. *Process review and planning* constitute a final element of the group; they enable leaders to examine their effectiveness, monitor the consistency of the protocol, and support each other. For example, after each session, a process note taker gives feedback to leaders in a "wrap-up" meeting.

Preparation

The psychoeducational groups require about a month of preparation. We believe that clinic staff members should be actively involved in the groups. Client attendance is better when staff members are part of the group counseling activities. Thus, leaders orient the clinic staff to the structure, content, and process of the groups. Part of the group preparation may also involve scheduling a demonstration workshop for staff members or inviting a clinic staff member to colead a group. The groups seem to benefit from having a diverse leader team. A professional with advanced training in behavioral science can provide therapeutic skills as well as adherence to protocol. Paraprofessionals in advanced stages of recovery help increase the level of trust and build group cohesion.

Client recruitment is straightforward. Clients are invited into the group and given a written description of the group's objectives, time commitment, and schedule of sessions. Clients are more likely to attend if they receive written and telephone reminders of the meetings for each session. Group leaders can also consider posting flyers around the clinic that describe counseling groups and their time schedule. Leaders might also consider spending time in the waiting room area on the day of each session to remind clients personally of their group counseling session. Clients seem to appreciate the personal and individual contact through these reminders.

Educational Tools and Supplies

A fair amount of didactic information is presented; doing this is easier with the use of a videocassette recorder and TV monitor, flip chart, or blackboard. Since the group teaches condom use and needle-cleaning skills, condom use and needle-cleaning kits and checklists (see Table 7.1) should be available. The checklists are used to train people in systematically completing each of the steps involved in correct condom use and needle sterilization. These checklists provide the learner with immediate feedback on his or her performance. In addition, clients receive "survival" kits, which include an assortment of condoms, bleach, spermicidal gel with nonoxynol-9, and dental dams, to take home and demonstrate to a friend between sessions.

Practitioners may wish to revise the checklists for needle sterilization and condom use to reflect the current recommendations in their communities. We developed ours by consulting with local experts in health education and outreach to drug users. Several organizations have collaborated on these checklists, attempting to provide a consistent message to drug users in San Francisco about how to clean their needles.

TABLE 7.1. Needle Cleaning and Condom Use Checklist

Checklist for Needle Sterilization Demonstration

__ 1. Filled container with bleach.
__ 2. Filled syringe completely with bleach.
__ 3. Emptied bleach from syringe into another container.
__ 4. Filled syringe completely with bleach for a second time.
__ 5. Emptied bleach from syringe into another container.
__ 6. Filled another container with water.
__ 7. Filled syringe completely with water.
__ 8. Emptied water from syringe into another container.
__ 9. Filled syringe completely with water a second time.
__ 10. Emptied water from syringe into another container.

Checklist for the Correct Condom Use Demostration

__ 1. Opened condom package without tearing condom.
__ 2. Applied lube to inside of condom.
__ 3. Pinched tip and rolled condom down.
__ 4. Applied lube on outside of condom (and partner).
__ 5. After ejaculation, held base of phallus and removed phallus with condom.
__ 6. Disposed of condom without spilling fluids.

In developing these recommendations for needle sterilization we encountered several points of debate, which may have been resolved differently in other communities. Some communities may recommend using a bleach-and-water solution rather than full-strength bleach (Steps 2 and 4), because the virucidal ability will not be much less, and there will be less tendency to deteriorate the plastic and rubber in the syringe. However, we strongly emphasize the step of filling the syringe *completely* with bleach (Steps 2 and 4) and water (Steps 7 and 9); this seems to be the most frequent mistake in skills demonstrations. Other groups may also recommend a "soak cycle" in the instructions, allowing the bleach to remain in a filled syringe for a specific length of time. In some communities, rubbing alcohol may be recommended instead of bleach.

The condom use checklist may be modified also. The points of contention as they were developed surrounded Steps 1, 2, and 4. Subjects seldom had trouble opening the packet (Step 1), so it did not often need much emphasis in skill-building sessions. Step 2 is important, but too much lubricant can lead to the condom's slipping off the penis during actual intercourse. Likewise, after the checklist was completed, some studies came out indicating that some spermicidal gels create vaginal irritation, so Step 4 (applying lubricant to the exterior of the condom) may be modified in some communities or with certain spermicides. Step 5 (removing the phallus without spilling fluids) and Step 6 (disposing of condom without spilling fluids) were readily accepted by participants, and most had not thought much about these issues before the training. Consequently, we strongly recommend that Steps 5 and 6 be included in revisions of the checklist for condom use.

An important educational tool is a chart explaining the concept of levels of defense against AIDS in terms of drug use (see top of Figure 1.1, Chapter 1). With this chart, leaders explain that abstinence (i.e., not using drugs at all) is the best, most complete defense against getting AIDS through drug use. Leaders acknowledge that despite this, not everyone is always abstinent. Therefore, as the chart illustrates, the next best way to defend against AIDS involves not injecting drugs. Since some people are unable to consistently avoid injection drug use, the chart indicates that the next level of defense involves not sharing "works" (i.e., syringes, cookers, and cottons). Finally, the leaders state that if clients do share their works, the only defense left between clients and AIDS is to clean needles before using them.

A second chart that describes the levels of defense against AIDS in terms of sexual behavior is another helpful educational tool to use in psychoeducational groups (see bottom of Figure 1.1, Chapter 1). A leader explains that abstinence is the best possible way to avoid contracting AIDS through sexual behavior. Since abstinence is probably unrealistic for many clients, the next best defense against AIDS is monogamy. Leaders remind clients that if they are engaging in risky needle use, then a monogamous relationship provides no protection for a sexual partner. Finally, the last level of defense between the client and AIDS is condom use.

First Session: Introducing the Concepts

"Are bruises which do not heal a sign of AIDS?"

"Can dialysis screen out the virus?"

These are the kinds of questions that leaders can expect in the first session of an AIDS prevention group. The leaders welcome the clients and establish ground rules. They ask clients not to reveal the results of any prior HIV antibody tests. Reasons for not disclosing serostatus include avoiding nonsupportive behaviors of group members toward the seropositive member and preventing seropositive clients from feeling alienated from seronegative members during group sessions. To tap personal feelings regarding the epidemic, leaders ask group members whether they know someone who has AIDS or has died from AIDS.

Segments from a videotape, *Conversations about AIDS and Drug Abuse* (Sorensen, Gibson, & Boudreaux, 1988a), make the epidemic real for clients by showing drug users with HIV disease speaking about how they learned of their diagnosis. The first session also informs clients about the factual aspects of AIDS and defines the medical terminology associated with the illness. Leaders explain the link between drug use and AIDS, and educate clients about how drug use and needle sharing put injection drug users at risk for AIDS.

Leaders ask clients what they think is risky in terms of drug use, and list these behaviors on one side of a chart under the heading "High risk." Leaders then ask clients how to decrease each high-risk activity. The chart depicting the levels of defense against AIDS in drug use is used to teach clients how to think about risky needle use practices and prevention strategies that can lower risk.

"It's easy to say, 'OK, just this once,' and not clean your needle. I am not going to lie. . . I do practice bad things."

"They had a big bleach bottle and filled a little one so they could go into the bedroom to use. Rigs all marked with initials . . . people are so scared."

As the quotations above illustrate, needle cleaning is an important part of AIDS prevention efforts. In Session 1 the leaders conduct a needle-cleaning demonstration. Each client subsequently teams up with a partner to practice the procedure. Clients take turns being in learning and teaching roles. The needle-cleaning checklist (see Table 7.1) provides each client with specific feedback on needle-cleaning skills. The first session concludes by eliciting and discussing clients' reactions to the group and by assigning homework. Clients are asked to inquire and report about how someone in their social circle cleans needles. Leaders summarize information covered in the session and mention some of the barriers to a less risky lifestyle.

Second Session: Sexual Behavior

Leaders begin the second session by welcoming participants and praising them for returning to the group and taking control of their lives by learning about AIDS. Homework from Session 1 is reviewed, and the leaders set the stage to discuss the ways that AIDS can be contracted and transmitted through unsafe sexual behavior. Various sexual activities are discussed, and clients are asked to comment on whether specific sexual practices are safe, possibly safe, or unsafe. Leaders elicit ideas from clients to explore ways to decrease risk. Concepts such as abstinence, monogamy, and other safe sexual practices are described. Barriers to safe sexual practices are elicited from group members, and leaders gently confront clients' resistances:

"Well, if my partner didn't want me to use a condom, I would probably have sex with her anyway if she was a 'nice girl.'"

"I have a friend. . . . [Her man] doesn't know she chips [injects only occasionally], so using condoms might give it away."

AIDS prevention supplies (such as condoms and spermicidal gel) are discussed by the group, as well as alternatives to intercourse (such as massage and mutual masturbation). In addition, the chart describing the levels of defense against AIDS through sexual activity is used to teach clients about altering HIV risk. A group leader then demonstrates the six-step procedure of correct condom use (using a wax phallus), and clients are asked to practice it in pairs. Clients begin by assigning themselves to a learner or teacher role. The client in the teacher role not only demonstrates how to use a condom, but also verbalizes each step in the process. The client in the learner role records each completed step on the condom use checklist. Clients switch roles after practicing the procedure twice.

Clients are then asked to practice introducing condom use to their sexual partners. Group leaders give pointers on negotiation skills, and participants role-play various scenarios. In one such exercise, one person proposes condom use, while the partner declines. Clients explore the possible positive arguments that may help persuade the reluctant sexual partner. Participants also practice responses to rationalizations that may be given by partners for no condom use. Leaders model assertive responses to the uncooperative or coercive sexual partner.

Group leaders assign homework that asks clients to experiment with different types of condoms and to make condoms a part of their sex play. "Survival kits," which contain condoms, spermicidal gel with nonoxynol-9, and dental dams, are passed out to group members. Clients are also assigned the homework task of talking with a sexual partner about condom use, and listing rationalizations and counterarguments for not using condoms. Session 2 is concluded by having clients rehearse condom use and needle-cleaning procedures, and by reviewing risky sexual and needle use practices.

Third Session: HIV Testing and Review

"I would never use that brand of condoms because they bunch up and they are too thin. Heavy-duty condoms are best."

"I threw my condoms away. They were hard to put on, they were too tight, and they didn't stay on."

Group leaders begin this session by discussing the homework assigned in the second session. Needle cleaning, condom use procedures, and factual knowledge about AIDS are reviewed. Group leaders help reinforce new knowledge by structuring quiz-like questions on material presented in the first two sessions. A highlight of the third session is the discussion of HIV antibody testing. Clients are shown a videotape such as *AIDS Antibody Testing at Alternative Test Sites* (Adair Films, 1985). Group leaders explore members' reactions to the video, and they lead a discussion about the advantages and disadvantages of testing. Clients are told not to reveal their serostatus while in the group, but leaders elicit members' concerns and ambivalence about antibody testing. Members are encouraged to think about what impact a positive test result might have on their lives. Group leaders neither encourage nor discourage antibody testing; rather, they provide information so that clients can make their own informed decisions. Leaders also provide clients with guidelines about how often to test, and inform them about the availability of testing through the drug treatment program and other community agencies. The following quotations illustrate common client reactions to antibody testing:

"If I got a positive antibody test I would purposely overdose."

"What's the point of being reinfected? If you got it, you got it!"

"I had to take the antibody test because I want to lead a normal, healthy life."

In bringing the 6-hour intervention to a close, leaders assist clients in reviewing condom and needle use and negotiation skills, as well as in repeating the role-playing exercises. Leaders summarize the key points covered during the three sessions, and invite clients to voice their reactions to the AIDS prevention groups. Participants generally make positive comments at this time, as the following quotes illustrate:

"I really liked this group. This is the first time I've been able to talk about this—to spill my guts."

"I learned a lot about sexual practices from the group. I knew the [injection] drug information, and the group taught me more than the pamphlets did."

"I thought I knew everything there was to know. I learned a lot

more. If there was anything it did, it was to raise my awareness. It will help me talk about it more."

CONDUCTING GROUPS WITH DIFFERENT DRUG USER POPULATIONS

Residential Treatment Programs

"Since our treatment program requires volunteer work, we can do work that is related to AIDS. We should take the information we have gotten in group and share it with [injection] drug users in detox and methadone maintenance programs."

Our psychoeducational AIDS prevention groups were created initially for clients in residential drug treatment. These clients did not actively rehearse condom use or needle-cleaning skills. The staff of the treatment program was opposed to the teaching of needle-cleaning skills, because it seemed to contradict the program's recovery orientation. Since clients in residential treatment, especially in the later phase of recovery, may demonstrate better adjustment and sounder ego function, these clients may be amenable to and interested in using their group counseling experience to educate other injection users about AIDS prevention. We have modified the group sessions accordingly and encouraged clients in residential drug treatment to participate as "change agents" in their community. Clients are encouraged to volunteer in agencies serving people with AIDS, as well as to engage in public speaking at churches, schools, and Narcotics Anonymous (NA) meetings. Clients are also encouraged to start an association for recovering addicts, and to represent the needs of injection drug users through social action by writing to the city council and becoming better informed about city and national politics.

Outpatient Detoxification Programs

Since clients in outpatient detoxification programs are much less reliable in keeping appointments or staying in treatment, when we conduct groups with them we mass the intervention into two sessions rather than three. The first session is 4 hours long and the second session 2 hours. We have not tried a single 6-hour session because it would eliminate the benefit of homework assignments between sessions. The homework provides a chance for the workshop to reach beyond clients to their friends and sexual partners, so we have chosen to keep it. In the 4-

hour session the leaders provide lunch, which keeps participants from wandering away from the sessions and adds to the social interaction.

Multicultural Aspects: Ethnic, Sexual, and Minorities

"A friend of mine thinks that AIDS is an FBI plot to get rid of all the dope fiends and minorities and homosexuals in the country."

The cultural diversity among injection drug users presents unique challenges to service providers attempting the group approach. Incorporating multicultural strategies becomes essential in the design, development, and execution of the interventions, especially in relation to AIDS. A group session may include multiethnic and multiracial populations, gays and lesbians, transvestites and transsexuals, persons in the sex industry, single parents, pregnant addicts, persons at various stages of acculturation and English-language acquisition, and different generational groups. Many injection drug users are of some combination of these different groups and lifestyles, which further complicates the multicultural issues facing the service provider. To be effective, AIDS prevention efforts need to reflect sensitivity to these cultural differences. It is unreasonable to expect clinical competence in working with all of these groups, but the service provider can be aware of and knowledgeable about the psychosocial and cultural differences among such groups.

In conducting AIDS prevention sessions, the multicultural aspects become an integral part of the group dynamics. For instance, many members of ethnic and racial minorities develop a keen sense of skepticism and suspicion when the government directs messages to them, ordering them to change their behavior or stating that their group is "at the highest risk" for some health epidemic. Leaders can expect discussion in the group session to center around the politics of AIDS and the feeling that this may be a federal law enforcement plot to eliminate undesirables. Another issue to expect is the expression of homophobic attitudes or moral judgment toward different lifestyles. Insensitive statements can alienate group members and divert the focus of the group from AIDS. Consequently, in preparing to conduct AIDS prevention groups, the facilitator needs to be well versed in the multicultural issues and attitudinal barriers.

In addition, while maintaining group cohesion and a balanced discussion, the group facilitator must keep the purpose and protocol of the group in focus. Some hints for group facilitators may help simplify this complex process. First, a facilitator should keep the group focused on the

AIDS issues and risk factors, and note that the information applies to everybody. The history of political oppression and its possible applications to the politics of AIDS should be acknowledged, as should the fact that it is OK and sometimes healthy to be suspicious. However, the participants cannot discount or minimize the threat of AIDS: Regardless of politics, this is the AIDS reality. Second, racial and homophobic tensions directed at individuals should be treated in the same way as any other type of interpersonal tension. Respect for group members is critical, and participants who cannot tolerate different group members may not be appropriate for group interventions. Third, facilitators should make the groups fun. They should use humor to disarm defenses, and keep the group lively. For example, we have begun groups by playing a taped "AIDS Rap" song. In leading the sessions, a variety of teaching methods can be used to communicate information and reinforce social change. When pairing group members for the exercises, facilitators might try having contests to see which partner can do the exercise faster or can do it within a certain time frame. We have seen condom "relay races" used in large-group settings. These exercises can be fun, and they reinforce the learning of skills. Fourth, a facilitator should be watchful for group members who are silent. Silence does not necessarily mean consent, agreement, or understanding; nor does it necessarily signal lack of interest, negativism, apathy, or boredom. Silence may be a sign of respect toward a facilitator, or it may be combined with misunderstanding, particularly among the less acculturated group members.

One advantage in working with injection drug users is their tendency to be frank and bold about how they feel. Some groups can be very lively, highly interactive, and stimulating. Encouraging the group members to be open and candid in their remarks may help them feel connected with each other and keep the process meaningful. The combination of a stimulating and enjoyable time with an atmosphere of respect for the multicultural diversity within the group has the basic elements of a positive group process in AIDS prevention with injection drug users. Groups can also be run for selected populations (e.g., gay couples, women, or long-term drug users) and tailored to their special concerns.

Integration into Clinic Operations

"The poster in the detox clinic that encourages users to clean their needles makes me want to fix because the stuff looks good."

"I have noticed that AIDS prevention posters don't tell us to clean cookers and not share water. This information should be given out."

Evaluation of current psychoeducational AIDS prevention counseling groups suggests that counseling does have an impact on clients by changing their attitudes about AIDS and some of the behaviors that put them at risk. Unfortunately, some of the positive changes from the counseling fade after about 3 months, so the future direction of psychoeducational groups will explore strategic ways to help clients maintain the changes made with group counseling. The urgency of preventing relapse to unsafe HIV-transmitting behavior is an emerging issue (Des Jarlais, Tross, Abdul-Quader, Kouzzi, & Friedman, 1989b), but relapse prevention has been of concern to the substance abuse field for some time (Marlatt & Gordon, 1985). Future program planning can explore how group leaders might instruct clinic staff members at different types of drug treatment programs in how to review key AIDS prevention strategies with clients. Group leaders might instruct treatment staffers who provide individual counseling and methadone dosing in setting up brief review sessions for high-risk injection drug users. Leaders might also train drug program counselors in condom use and needle-cleaning skills, so that clients can review these skills in their individual counseling sessions. In addition, leaders might instruct drug treatment programs in creating an on-site "prevention clinic" so that clients can learn to monitor their own risk for AIDS. If AIDS risk assessment procedures are made interesting enough to clients, some clients may be eager to learn whether their lifestyle is at high, medium, or low risk for AIDS. Self-assessment tools for clients might be another strategy for encouraging clients to remember what they learned in group counseling.

Group leaders might also institute periodic telephone "checkups" and arrange for "survival kits" to be mailed out (at regular intervals) to group participants. Sponsors from NA might be instructed in AIDS prevention techniques, and then they might be invited to pair up with group members who are having difficulty with modifying their AIDS risk level. Psychoeducational counseling groups are effective in decreasing clients' risk for AIDS, but many strategies need development and testing to maintain the gains clients make with this AIDS prevention method.

FUTURE DEVELOPMENT OF THE GROUP APPROACH

The group approach has also been successful in changing the risk behaviors of gay men who were not identified as drug users (Kelly et al., 1989). The group approach among gay men in San Francisco has been credited with changing high risk behavior and in slowing the spread of HIV. In-home groups facilitated by the grassroots "Stop AIDS" movement worked through personal networks to mobilize men to help each other prevent infection and to build community support (Puckett & Bye, 1987). Injection drug users are very different from groups of largely middle-class gay men, but the group approach nonetheless may have a significant impact among them as well.

Additional research is underway with drug-using subjects. *The experimental rigor and evidence of the efficacy of many programs vary* (somewhat inversely), with most outcomes reflecting improved knowledge, attitudes, or intentions rather than changed behaviors. Several studies nonetheless report behavioral changes as well. The study by Schilling et al. (1989a, in press) found that subjects in a skill-building group were more likely than information-only controls to carry condoms. Magura et al. (1989c, in press) found that subjects in peer education groups reported greater condom use. Our research team found that outpatients in both methadone maintenance and detoxification improved in behavioral demonstrations of skills in sterilizing syringes and using condoms.

In general, the emerging results indicate that the group approach has promise as an AIDS prevention technique in treatment programs. The approach is better than providing information alone. However, the modest outcomes point out the difficulty of altering high-risk behavior. The studies will require peer review, publication of results, and further development. If their results warrant further work, later collaborative studies may incorporate the most powerful aspects of these interventions in controlled, multisite investigations. Meanwhile, they serve as a basis for further AIDS prevention efforts.

ACKNOWLEDGMENTS

This chapter reflects contributions of a larger research team than the author list reflects. We particularly appreciate the contributions of David R. Gibson to the measurement of effects; Roland Dumontet to the content of the small-group sessions; and Carma Heitzmann to coordination of the psychoeducational groups. The staff and patients of Substance Abuse Services, San Francisco General Hospital, and of Walden House, Inc., in San Francisco, deserve special thanks.

Chapter 8

Individual Counseling

DAVID R. GIBSON
JANE LOVELLE-DRACHE

The brief counseling described in this chapter has an important practical aim: to reduce behaviors that put injection drug users at risk for AIDS. The brief format of the counseling (50–60 minutes) balances the need for intensive interventions to change behavior with the need for a cost-effective strategy of reaching large numbers of drug users. Risk reduction interventions must be practical if they are to reach a significant proportion of the population at risk. Expensive and time-consuming interventions such as individual psychotherapy cannot contribute significantly to AIDS prevention efforts. At the same time, widespread distribution of leaflets and warnings in the electronic print media, although helpful, are probably not sufficient to change the behavior of individuals at risk. The brief counseling we have designed is a non-labor-intensive intervention that provides drug users with basic current information about AIDS transmission, while helping them to develop confidence in confronting high-risk situations. If effective, the counseling sessions could be widely disseminated to drug treatment programs at low cost and with minimal staff training.

We begin this chapter by reviewing the theoretical principles that have guided the design of the counseling sessions and describing how these principles have been implemented. After briefly covering preparation for the counseling sessions, we describe them in some detail. The counseling sessions are intended to be flexibly structured, and to be interactive rather than didactic. They are designed to involve the drug users in problem solving, in situations where they are tempted to engage in high-risk practices.

THEORETICAL RATIONALE

The theoretical framework that guided the design of the counseling sessions is the AIDS risk reduction model (ARRM; Catania, Kegeles, &

Coates, 1990), which has been described in Chapter 5. The three-stage model is an effort to describe the process by which people attempt to change sexual behaviors related to HIV transmission. Catania and his colleagues note that with minor modifications, the model may also be applied to other HIV-related behaviors, particularly those involved with injection drug use. The focus of the ARRM is on psychological and social factors involved in the labeling of high-risk behaviors as problematic (Stage 1), in the development of commitment to changing those behaviors (Stage 2), and in the seeking and enactment of solutions directed at reducing high-risk activities (Stage 3). These factors have been discussed in some detail in Chapter 5. Here we describe how they have influenced the design of the counseling sessions.

1. *Knowledge about HIV risk transmission* is essential if a drug user is to see his or her behavior as problematic (Stage 1). In the counseling sessions, we aim to provide accurate, essential information about how AIDS is contracted.

2. *Susceptibility* is also important to recognition of high-risk behaviors. To increase perceived susceptibility, we provide drug users with information that brings home their vulnerability, including the fact that many of their drug-using peers are infected with HIV.

3. *Response efficacy* (perceived benefit of risk reduction practices) is enhanced by thoroughly discussing recommended guidelines to reduce risk, in which the drug user's objections to the guidelines are carefully considered. Alternate risk reduction practices are then discussed. Response efficacy is necessary if the drug user is to commit himself or herself to behavior change (Stage 2 of the ARRM).

4. *Self-efficacy* is a key variable in risk reduction. We have seen in Chapter 4 that self-efficacy is strongly and negatively correlated with needle sharing, and is also correlated positively to condom use. It appears to be important primarily at the commitment and enactment stages of behavior change (Stages 2 and 3). In the counseling sessions, we promote self-efficacy with problem solving designed to help drug users anticipate and deal with situations in which they may be tempted to share needles or engage in unprotected sex.

5. *Communication skill* is closely related to self-efficacy and is important at the enactment stage (Stage 3). Communication skills are developed by rehearsing and role-playing conversational gambits that drug users can use in negotiating safe needle practices. We also help drug users to deal with resistance that they are likely to encounter from friends and partners.

6. *Perceived severity* is heightened by discussing sequelae of HIV infection and showing drug users a photograph of a person in the end

stages of the disease. McKusick, Horstman, and Coates (1985b) found that among gay men, having a clear mental image of AIDS deterioration was one of the strongest predictors of risk reduction. Perceived severity may lead to a heightened level of anxiety. According to Catania et al. (1990, p. 65), persistent anxiety may play a role in movement from one stage of behavior change to the next.

7. *Social support* is difficult to build in one-on-one counseling sessions. However, it may be possible if the counselor is a recovered drug user or other "streetwise" person who is viewed as a peer or role model. Also, it is possible in the counseling sessions to encourage drug users to become change agents in their social group.

OVERVIEW

The protocol for the counseling calls for two sessions: an initial session lasting 50–60 minutes, and a 10- to 15-minute follow-up session (usually occurring 10–14 days after the first session). Both sessions are one-on-one encounters between a counseling staff member and a drug user.

As currently designed, the brief counseling sessions have three components: (1) a brief didactic presentation of essential factual information about routes of HIV transmission and risk reduction; (2) problem solving of situations in which the drug user is tempted to engage in high-risk practices; and (3) demonstration of recommended procedures for using condoms and sterilizing needles and syringes. The key feature of the counseling sessions is the problem solving, in which the counselor and the drug user review situations in which the drug user is tempted to engage in high-risk activities, and together they develop a risk reduction plan tailored to the individual drug user's needs.

PREPARATION FOR THE COUNSELING

Before attempting the counseling, a counselor needs to thoroughly review the treatment manual (obtainable from David R. Gibson). In delivering the counseling sessions, the counselor will have available a looseleaf binder of visual aids to cue issues that need to be covered. The visual aids are both a prop and a guide to the initial counseling session, which covers the issues under three main headings (basic facts, drugs, and sex). The visual aids free the counselor of the task of remembering issues that need to be covered. Within the three main headings, the issues can be addressed in any order. The intent is to encourage a flexible and spontaneous discussion of the drug user's problems, at the same time insuring that all issues are addressed. The counselor should be sufficiently familiar with all of the issues that they can be dealt with comfortably as they come up naturally in the course of a counseling session.

In addition to the binder of visual aids, other materials needed include a "Plans to Reduce Risk" form, which is used in the problem solving, and a demonstration kit containing items needed for the condom and needle-cleaning demonstration (condoms, foams, syringe, bleach, water, etc.). Drug users also receive a "safe sex" kit and a 32-page handbook that covers the high points of the counseling session; the handbook also includes helpful information, such as where to seek drug treatment or buy condoms. The handbook presents many of the same materials that appear in the binder of visual aids, and is designed to reinforce what the drug user has gained from the counseling.

INITIAL SESSION (50–60 MINUTES)

The initial session has three parts: a 5- to 10-minute review of essential factual information; a 15- to 20-minute discussion of issues related to AIDS and substance abuse; and a 20- to 25-minute discussion of AIDS and sexual practices. The issues surrounding sexual practices tend to be more complicated and usually require more discussion. However, the counselor should focus on whatever issues are most problematic for a given drug user, briefly covering those that seem less central.

The counselor begins the initial session by describing the aims of the counseling. These are to provide the drug user with essential factual information, to find out how he or she is coping, and to solve problems that may be getting in the way of risk reduction.

In presenting the basic facts about AIDS, the counselor may want to acknowledge that "most of these things you probably know, but we want to cover them all just to make sure." The eight basic facts covered have been adapted from those compiled by the editors of the Johns Hopkins quarterly *Population Reports* (Johns Hopkins, 1986). They include information about how the disease is spread and about how it can be prevented. We have opted for a minimal presentation of essential information. Too much information can overwhelm drug users, making it difficult for them to see the forest for the trees. Also, it is important early in the session to engage a drug user in actively thinking about his or her problems. Too much didactic presentation has the tendency to put the drug user in a passive mode. The material should therefore be covered quickly. The counselor, however, should be alert to any confusion on the drug user's part, and take time to answer carefully any questions that may come up.

Next, the counselor should discuss the course of HIV disease, beginning with infection and asymptomatic carrier status and progressing to diagnosis and clinical manifestations of AIDS. Our binder of visual aids includes the cartoon "How People Get AIDS" (commissioned from San Francisco cartoonist Lloyd Dangle; see Figure 8.1). The cartoon depicts different ways people can become infected with HIV, as well as possible sequelae of infection (AIDS-related complex [ARC], opportunistic infections such as pneumocystis pneumonia and Kaposi's sarcoma, etc.). The object is to help drug users quickly assess their susceptibility to AIDS. In reviewing the cartoon, the counselor should provide information about how widespread HIV infection is in a community, and point out that most people who are infected can look forward to serious medical problems.

At this point, the counselor may wish to pause and ask whether the drug user knows or knew anyone with AIDS. The binder of visual aids contains a photograph of a seriously ill AIDS patient, to give drug users a clear mental picture of the potential severity of HIV illness. This may be particularly important in communities where few drug users have contracted AIDS. A discussion of the more common HIV infections (see above) is recommended to bring home the seriousness of being infected.

For some drug users, this frank discussion of HIV disease will understandably occasion anxiety. They may not have considered the degree to which their behavior has put them at risk, or may not have adequately grasped the severity of HIV disease. In order to bind the anxiety (which otherwise may be disabling), the counselor needs to reassure a drug user that there are things he or she can do to avoid contracting the disease.

This observation is a natural lead-in to a discussion of how the drug user can manage risk, which takes up the balance of the counseling session. In this discussion, the counselor needs to engage the drug user as a full partner, at the same time keeping the agenda of the counseling session clearly in mind. We recommend that, within the sections dealing with drug use and sexual practices, topics be covered in any order that seems comfortable and natural and is focused on the individual drug user's particular problems. This requires some agility, but often becomes easier as the drug user warms to the subject. One technique we have found useful is to encourage the drug user to play the role of an expert from whom the counselor has as much to learn as vice versa (this is certainly the case).

AIDS and Injection Drug Use

Discussion of what drug users can do to reduce risk should be kept simple. We recommend that risk reduction be presented in terms of "levels of defense" (see Chapter 1, top of Figure 1.1). The following simple for-

HOW PEOPLE GET AIDS
SHOOTING DRUGS WITH USED NEEDLES
RESULTS OF BECOMING INFECTED:
-UNSAFE SEX WITH AN INFECTED PERSON.
LUCKY ME!
NO SYMPTOMS.
THE SYMPTOMS:
SWOLLEN GLANDS
NIGHT SWEATS
THRUSH MOUTH
EXCESSIVE WEIGHT LOSS
DIARRHEA
FATIGUE
???
I CAN FEEL GREAT
FOR 7 YEARS OR MORE...
ARC
AIDS
ILLNESS CONTINUES, BECOMING SEVERE.
KAPOSI'S SARCOMA
PNEUMONIA
TOXOPLASMOSIS
AIDS DEMENTIA
...AND STILL BE ABLE TO SPREAD THE VIRUS.
???
???
©1988 DANGLE
AIDS
1 TO 2 YRS
SO I SHOULDN'T SHARE NEEDLES
OR HAVE SEX WITHOUT CONDOMS.
I'VE GOT TO DO MY BEST TO STAY HEALTHY.

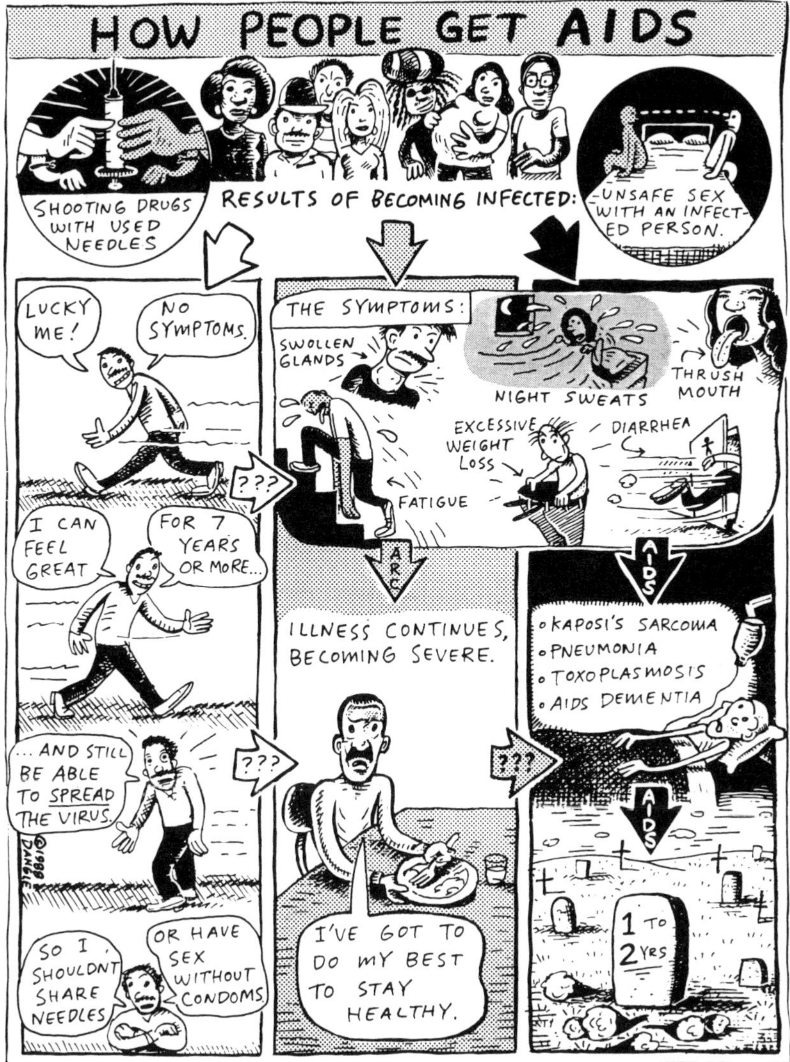

FIGURE 8.1. Methods of HIV transmission. The cartoon is by Lloyd Dangle and is reprinted with his permission.

mula is easily grasped: "Don't use drugs; if you must, don't share needles or other paraphernalia; if you must share, clean your equipment between uses."

With each of these injunctions, it is possible to explore concrete steps the drug user can take. In relation to giving up drugs, it is important to explore the drug user's willingness to accept drug treatment (methadone maintenance, inpatient residential treatment, detoxification, Narcotics Anonymous). Because the demand for drug treatment often exceeds the supply, drug users need to be prepared for obstacles they are likely to encounter, including being put on a waiting list. Such obstacles should not provide an excuse for failing to follow through. It may be helpful to remind the drug user of the longer-term benefits of drug treatment, one of the most important of which is risk reduction. Similarly, the barriers to inpatient treatment (e.g., separation from spouse/lover/friends) need to be acknowledged but weighed against the drug user's longer-term interests. Practical advice about where to apply for drug treatment should be offered. We provide drug users with a list of referrals that includes drug treatment programs.

Next, especially for drug users unwilling to consider treatment, the difficulties of not sharing injection equipment need to be explored. It is helpful at this point to discuss the drug user's drug injection patterns. We have seen in Chapter 5 that drug users who inject drugs in public places are much more likely to share equipment. We recommend that active drug users inject drugs at home, where a supply of sterile needles can be kept, along with disinfectant for cleaning injection equipment. Having "guest works" available for friends may also reduce the temptation to share equipment. It is also helpful to explore drug users' access to sterile syringes through a syringe exchange, pharmacist, diabetic friend, or street dealer. Would a drug user have difficulty refusing to share equipment with a friend, or trouble broaching the issue of needle hygiene with others? What are some of the comfortable ways of doing this?

The counselor needs to be alert to rationalizations. "I only shoot up with my old man/lady" is a common excuse. The pitfalls of such rationalizations need to be acknowledged in a nonthreatening manner.

The "Plans to Reduce Risk" form (see Figure 8.2 for a sample) can be produced at this point. The point of the form is to review situations in which the drug user engages in high-risk behavior (when depressed, in withdrawal, without "works"). The counselor and user can then apply problem solving to practical difficulties, and alternatives to high-risk behaviors can be discussed. It is particularly useful to help a drug user to anticipate situations where he or she would be tempted to share injection equipment, so that the drug user can avoid such situations in the future. Injecting drugs at home, where one has access to sterile equipment or disinfectant and running water, is an obvious possibility. It may also be useful to discuss how withdrawal symptoms can distort judgment. Many drug users tell us that in such circumstances they simply don't care. One technique for countering this kind of apathy is to have a drug user recall his or her emotional reaction to the death of a friend lost to AIDS, or to imagine what having AIDS would be like.

Risky Things I've Done	When I've Done Them	Plans to Avoid Doing Them
Used someone else's works	On the street didn't have my own	Shoot up at home always have works handy
Have sex with strangers	High on Crack	Seek treatment for addiction

FIGURE 8.2. Sample of a "Plans to Reduce Risk" form.

Demonstration of procedures for disinfecting needles serves the purpose of getting the drug user to begin to think actively about risk reduction. The simplicity of disinfection procedures can be quickly demonstrated. We recommend the San Francisco AIDS Foundation disinfection guidelines, which call for a syringe to be flushed twice with bleach, and then twice with water. (The needle should be removed from the syringes to avoid accidental needle sticks.) The drug user should be coached in demonstrating the proper procedure. It is important to work through any misgivings or difficulties that the drug user may have.

Before turning to sexual matters, it is useful to review the "Plans to Reduce Risk" form. Are the plans realistic? Can the drug user commit to following through on them? The counselor should suggest that the drug user review the plans and his or her progress at regular intervals (the form is part of the handbook that the drug user takes away from the session).

AIDS and Sexual Practices

Issues concerning sexual risk reduction closely parallel those having to do with drugs. Which level of defense a drug user should adopt with regard to sexual behavior will vary from person to person. Three quite different strategies of dealing with infection are abstinence, an exclusive relationship with an uninfected partner, and the practice of safe sex (particularly the consistent use of condoms).

With regard to abstinence, the obvious needs to be acknowledged—that is, abstinence may be difficult for most people. However, abstinence should certainly be considered as an option where one or both partners are infected. Even when properly used, condoms frequently fail; although condoms greatly reduce the risk of infection, the risk is probably still unacceptably high.

Monogamy is a second option, although its effectiveness depends critically on the degree of trust established between a drug user and his or her sexual partner. Whether trust can be sustained when one or both partners are actively using drugs is a matter that the drug user and the partner need to consider. A general guideline we have followed in working with drug users is to avoid hard-and-fast prescriptions that preclude drug users from making their own decisions. At the same time, we feel that it is important to be clear about the consequences of different choices.

The choice of monogamy as a risk reduction strategy requires that both the drug user and partner submit to antibody testing. Because up to 6 months may elapse between infection and development of immune response, the drug user and partner should practice safe sex until a second test can firmly establish the antibody status of both. Once antibody status has been established, neither partner should engage in high-risk behavior for this option to be effective.

A third option includes the various forms of safe sex, including the use of condoms. For most injection drug users, using condoms will be the preferred means of preventing infection from sex. We recommend, however, that the counselor review the safety of a variety of sexual practices, since the drug user may be reluctant to discuss less conventional practices. To encourage candor, it is best to assume a nonjudgmental, neutral attitude toward sexual practices. Using the "Plans to Reduce Risk" form, we recommend reviewing circumstances in which the drug user has engaged in high-risk practices (under the influence of drugs and alcohol, etc.). The counselor and user should apply problem solving to these situations, and together should develop a plan for changing to safe options. The salient issues for male drug users usually include the perception that condoms reduce sensation and interfere with the spontaneity of sex. We have sometimes found it effective to point out that anxiety about infecting a partner can get in the way of sexual enjoyment. It is also helpful to discuss how lubricants properly used can increase sensation, or how condoms can be eroticized by incorporating them into foreplay.

The salient issues for women frequently revolve around getting a male partner to accept or at least to try condoms. A number of ways of broaching the use of condoms should be discussed. The binder of visual aids lists a number of these, reprinted from the book *How to Get Your Lover to Use a Condom and Why You Should* (Breitman, Knutson, & Reed, 1987). It is helpful to discuss which of the "openers" a woman would be comfortable using with her partner, and to role-play how she plans to initiate the subject with her partner. If the drug user feels that she and her partner are unlikely to use condoms, other forms of safe sex should be discussed.

The visual aids contain a number of tips for using condoms, including the use of lubricants and spermicidal foams and jellies. The counselor should review the principal reasons why condoms fail (e.g., the use of oil-based lubricants, air bubbles that cause them to abrade, etc.). As with disinfection of syringes, it is helpful for the drug user to practice proper procedures for using condoms by putting a condom on a dildo or candle. If the drug user has never used condoms or seldom used them, this demonstration may help to lower resistance to their use. At the same time, some of the fine points of using condoms can be illustrated. It is helpful to encourage the drug user to experiment with the different condoms, foams, and jellies in the safe sex kit. Drug users who have not previously used condoms need to be advised that condoms require getting used to before they become a natural and pleasurable part of lovemaking.

The counseling sessions are currently being evaluated in a controlled trial with 300 heroin detoxification outpatients recruited to the project between December 1987 and June 1989. The drug users were interviewed prior to random assignment to experimental counseling or an information-only brochures condition. Follow-up interviews were conducted at 10 days and at 3 and 12 months after intervention to assess the impact of the counseling. Preliminary analysis of the follow-up data indicates a marked reduction in needle sharing among drug users who received the experimental counseling, as well as a substantial decrease in unprotected intercourse (from about 63% to 44% at the 12-month follow-up). However, similar reductions in needle sharing were also observed for the comparison group (which received educational brochures), and group differences in sexual practices beyond the 10-day follow-up were not statistically significant. Preliminary analysis of the 3-month follow-up data indicates that the counseling sessions may have at least a short-term impact. Drug users receiving the counseling reported greater perceived susceptibility, greater response efficacy, and somewhat greater sexual self-efficacy (Gibson, Lovelle-Drache, Derby, Garcia-Soto, & Sorensen, 1989a; Gibson, Wermuth, Lovelle-Drache, Ham, & Sorensen, 1989b).

SUPPLEMENTS TO THE COUNSELING SESSIONS

Follow-Up Counseling

The equivocal results just presented suggest the need for strengthening the impact of individual counseling sessions. Of particular importance is the necessity of preventing relapse to unsafe practices. Among a large sample of San Francisco gay men, for example, 17% of those who succeeded in reducing or eliminating the practice of unprotected anal intercourse later relapsed to this practice (Ekstrand, Stall, Coates, & McKusick, 1990). How to maintain low-risk behavior after initial behavior change has been the subject of some controversy. Marlatt and George (1989) argue that the cessation of problem behaviors may be governed by principles entirely different from those leading to maintenance of behavior change. The main difference appears to be that initiation of change is often the result of treatment that is externally administered, whereas maintenance of behaviors is left to the treatment client to "self-administer." As a consequence, Marlatt and George believe that treatment to prevent relapse to problem behaviors must include a component that is grounded in self-monitoring and self-management skills.

The problem-solving element of our experimental counseling sessions is designed specifically to provide drug users with the self-management skills needed for long-term behavior change. In a modest way (given the brief format of the counseling), we help drug users to anticipate and plan for situations in which they may be tempted to engage in high-risk practices. Problem solving has proven to be an effective technique in dealing with other problem behaviors (D'Zurilla & Nezu, 1982). For example, Supnick and Coletti (1984) found that the problem-solving component of a program to reduce relapse to smoking led to lower relapse rates among ex-smokers who attended the program.

The follow-up session to the initial 50- to 60-minute session is intended to designed specifically to further strengthen problem-solving skills. The follow-up session is not a "booster" session; that is, it is not "more of the same." Booster sessions have generally not proven to be effective in promoting long-term behavior change (Brownell, Marlatt, Lichtenstein, & Wilson, 1986). In the follow-up session, which lasts 10–15 minutes and occurs 2 weeks after the initial session, the counselor reviews the drug user's success (or lack thereof) in implementing the "Plans to Reduce Risk." The follow-up session provides an opportunity for fine-tuning problem-solving skills and for dealing with problems inadequately addressed in the initial session. The drug user's experiences in the interval become grist for discussion of the difficulty of implementing changes.

Antibody Testing

HIV testing is another potentially effective adjunct to counseling. In many cases, antibody testing may help to personalize issues surrounding high-risk behavior, and to bring home the drug user's susceptibility to disease. HIV testing may prompt the drug user to review his or her past behavior and to consider appropriate changes in that behavior. Studies are showing that learning one's antibody status may result in decreased risk behavior. A negative result may help to dispel anxiety or fatalism, or become the occasion for turning over a new leaf. Drug users who test positive for the HIV antibody may begin to consider how their behavior puts others at risk or endangers their own health (Dilley, Seymour , & Eya, 1987).

Coates et al. (1988) reviewed nine studies that examined whether gay men who had been tested for the AIDS antibody were more or less likely to engage in high-risk sexual practices. In six of the nine studies, including a survey of 1,000 men in the Baltimore–Washington area, the number reporting unprotected anal intercourse declined substantially. The reductions were somewhat more dramatic for men who received seropositive results. Three other studies did not find any significant reductions in high-risk practices as a result of receiving positive test results.

Three conference presentations (Casadonte, Des Jarlais, Smith, Novatt, & Herndal, 1986; Cox, Selwyn, Schoenbaum, O'Dowd, & Drucker, 1986; Marlink et al., 1987) suggest that HIV testing may also be helpful to injection drug users. In all three studies, there was evidence of lower levels of drug injection and/or sharing of injection equipment. In the Casadonte et al. study, being tested resulted in increased practice of safe sex. Although these studies are encouraging concerning the use of HIV testing to promote risk reduction, Des Jarlais (1988a) warns that there may be unpresented studies that did not find positive results.

We are currently evaluating a modification of the brief counseling protocol to examine the impact of the counseling when coupled with receipt of antibody test results. In this enhanced intervention, the test result serves as a point of departure for a discussion of risk reduction. In the experimental counseling sessions, drug users are encouraged to make sense of their test results by reviewing their past behavior. We have found it useful to make the connection between behavior and test results explicit. If a drug user tests negative, we reinforce whatever efforts have been made toward risk reduction. To the extent that the appropriate changes have not been made, we make a point of observing that luck is a very fickle commodity. It is important that a negative test not be interpreted as evidence of immunity.

If a drug user tests positive, past behavior may help to put the result in context, although any implication of blame should be avoided. Many drug users anticipate a positive result and seem to take it in stride (A. R. Moss, personal communication, 1990). A positive result eliminates uncertainty, allowing a drug user to focus on the increased need to protect health and avoid infecting others. The drug user should be encouraged to think about "What do I do now?" or "Where do I go from here?"

Social Support for Behavior Change

As noted earlier, a drawback of individual counseling sessions is the difficulty in building peer support for risk reduction. In this regard, group counseling, such as that described in Chapter 7, has a decided advantage; however, in groups it is difficult to focus on an individual's problems, and it may also be awkward to discuss intimate matters (particularly those related to sexuality).

One way in which we have attempted to address the shortcoming of individual counseling is to encourage drug users to think about how they become involved as change agents in their communities. The substantial reductions in high-risk sexual practices noted among gay men in San Francisco have been largely attributed to self-organization by the gay community (McKusick, Coates, & Morin, 1990). Although similar attempts among drug users have been less effective (Friedman, de Jong, & Des Jarlais, 1988), the substantial reduction in needle sharing found by Guydish, Abramowitz, Woods, Black, and Sorensen (1990a), among others, suggests that social influences may be responsible. We therefore encourage drug users to take the opportunity to engage their peers in discussion of risk reduction. At the conclusion of the initial counseling session, a drug user is asked to distribute wallet-size cards describing recommended procedures for disinfecting syringes and using condoms. The benefit of this includes not only a potential multiplier effect ("each one teach one"), but also reinforcement of whatever the drug user has gained from the counseling session by role-playing the issues with others.

Another way of offsetting the disadvantage of individual counseling is to employ indigenous community members as counselors. A recovered drug user, for example, may be well known in social circles of current users, which adds to his or her credibility. He or she may be viewed not only as a peer but perhaps also as a role model. Bandura (1990) observes that self-efficacy can be enhanced if people can observe others like them solving problems successfully. The use of streetwise outreach workers has been very effective in San Francisco in promoting the use of ordinary household bleach for disinfection of needles and syringes (Watters, 1987).

CONCLUSION

The preliminary data presented earlier suggest that even very brief counseling sessions may have a significant impact on attitudes and behaviors placing injection drug users at risk for AIDS. An advantage of individual counseling is that it can be tailored to a drug user's specific difficulties in making behavioral changes. The counselor can quickly determine where the drug user is in the change process and can intervene to speed that process along. Some drug users may not perceive the extent to which their behavior is a problem. For these, information and awareness of personal susceptibility may be needed to initiate change. Other drug users may be aware of their risk, but may have difficulty in developing commitment to enact these changes. For this latter group, problem solving to help anticipate and cope with high-risk situations may be more effective. As mentioned, problem solving has the advantage of developing self-management skills that can help to prevent relapse to unsafe practices long after initial behavior change. By helping a drug user anticipate and plan for high-risk situations, problem solving increases the chances that the drug user's response in such a situation will be a coping one. Problem solving may also be useful in identifying situations that can simply be avoided. For example, always having a supply of sterile needles available can greatly lessen the temptation to share injection equipment.

Chapter 9

Reaching and Counseling Women Sexual Partners

LAURIE A. WERMUTH
REBECCA L. ROBBINS
KYUNG-HEE CHOI
RANI EVERSLEY

Women sexual partners of injection drug users compose an epidemiological category, but they do not form a natural social group or community. Most are not on "the streets," as are some social circles of male drug users. Women partners of drug-injecting men may have a similar type of AIDS risk, but their social and interpersonal circumstances are varied, as are the cultural frameworks that give meaning to their sexual relationships and their ideas about using condoms. Although urban underclass minority women make up the majority of this population, some middle-class women also have partners who inject drugs. Many women are unaware of their sexual partners' drug injecting, and consequently are unaware of their HIV risk. Other women are secretive about their partners' drug use and isolated from those who could encourage them to be cautious. For poor women, the immediate needs of obtaining food or shelter and caring for their children often overshadow worries about AIDS (Mays & Cochran, 1988; Murphy, 1988).

The percentage of reported AIDS cases among women attributed to heterosexual transmission is rising, increasing from 3% of cases diagnosed in 1988 to 34% in 1990. Much of this heterosexual spread comes from drug-injecting men (Centers for Disease Control [CDC], 1990a, 1991). Women's sexual risk for HIV is confounded by other factors. If women do not already inject drugs, they may be introduced to the practice by their male partners, and if they become infected and pregnant, their infants are at risk for perinatal AIDS. Women with sexual partners who are "in recovery" from drug use risk infection if their partners relapse to drug injecting and needle sharing. Women who have themselves injected drugs are additionally at risk for infection if they relapse to drug injection and needle sharing.

This chapter aims to familiarize readers with some of the problems facing the women sexual partners of drug-injecting men, and to suggest some activities that can help to lower their HIV risk. It first reviews selected literature on women and HIV risk, then describes methods for reaching women sexual partners of injection drug users. A model for individual counseling is then offered, followed by a description of the ways in which women cope with their risk, and an exploration of some clinical issues. The counseling model and description of coping strategies are based on a study of women sexual partners of male drug injectors in the San Francisco Bay Area.

WOMEN, AIDS RISK, AND CONSTRAINTS ON SELF-PROTECTION: A SELECTIVE REVIEW OF THE LITERATURE

All women are not equally at risk for AIDS. Risk profiles show that African-American and Hispanic women have a disproportionately high prevalence of AIDS (CDC, 1990a). Worth and Rodriguez (1987) found that among the Hispanic women they studied in the Lower East Side of New York City, the risk for infection was 11 times that found among white women. African-American women make up 12% of the U.S. female population, but 52% of the AIDS cases among women; Hispanic women make up 6% of the female population, but 20% of female AIDS cases (CDC, 1990a). By comparison, white women comprise 27% of the female AIDS cases and 79.5% of the female population (CDC, 1990a). Once a person is diagnosed with AIDS, the rate of mortality differs drastically by race, gender, and sexual orientation. Differences may be reflected in differential timing in seeking medical care, in recognition of the disease by practitioners, and also in differences in ability to fend off fatal illness. A New York City study found that the overall survival rate for African-American women at 1 year from diagnosis was 37%, as compared to 75% for white gay men (Rothenberg et al., 1987).

Becker and Joseph's (1988) review of behavior changes to prevent transmission of HIV revealed discrepancies in the adoption of condom use. For example, studies have found that 80% of prostitutes used condoms with their customers, but only 16% practiced safe sex with their husbands or boyfriends (CDC, 1987; Cohen, Alexander, & Wofsy, 1988). Women prostitutes who were addicted were less likely to be protected by even customers' use of condoms. This may reflect greater urgency in their trade as a result of the demands of addiction. Condom use among male heterosexual injectors appears to be low. Lewis, Watters, and Case's (1990) study of 149 male injection drug users in San Francisco with steady female partners found that 73% never used condoms and that 83% of the respondents had multiple partners.

Studies examining women's views about AIDS have found that many believe they are inherently safe from the disease, think they have nothing to learn about it, and therefore do not feel the need to change (Cohen, Hauer, & Wofsy, 1989; Evans, 1987). Worth and Rodriguez (1987) found that most of the young Hispanic women they interviewed in a New York neighborhood with a high prevalence of drug injection and AIDS did not realize their personal risk of contracting the disease. Among these sexually active teenage women, only a few understood that AIDS could be caught from their boyfriends. In Los Angeles, women interviewed believed African-Americans to be less at risk for AIDS than whites (Mays & Cochran, 1988).

Women at highest risk for AIDS are among the most disadvantaged in the United States. Factors that depress women's self-efficacy and constrain their ability to protect themselves include drug and alcohol use, poverty, cultural norms, gender roles, and sexuality issues. If they do not inject drugs themselves, women may be introduced to the practice by their male partners (Rosenbaum, 1981a; Zahn & Ball, 1974), or they may relapse to drug use or become susceptible to sexual transmission if their partners relapse. Women crack cocaine users are at especially high risk for HIV transmission, because they often trade sex for drugs or money with men who have relatively high rates of HIV infection (Weissman, Sowder, & Young, 1990).

Studies of poor and drug-dependent women paint a depressing picture regarding risk for HIV (M. T. Fullilove, Fullilove, Haynes, & Gross, 1990a; Cohen et al., 1989; M. T. Fullilove, 1988; Mays & Cochran, 1988; Mondanaro, 1987; Wofsy, 1987). Their life options are limited. They are often subject to violence, and their daily circumstances are stressful. Addicted women are largely unemployed; many have not completed high school. The majority are African-American or Hispanic. When asked to alter their sexual or drug use behavior, these women may experience further emotional discomfort in acknowledging the lack of power they have in their relationships, over their drug use, and in the daily risks they face. Addressing possible HIV risk may bring up a disturbing life history, disappointments, and feelings of self-blame. Our analysis of factors associated with acknowledgment of HIV risk in a sample of 77 women sexual partners of injection drug users found that employed women were seven times more likely than unemployed women to perceive themselves at risk (Wermuth, Choi, Ham, Falcone, & Hulley, 1991). It may be that some degree of control over one's daily life via monetary resources (however meager) makes it possible for women to address their risk for HIV infection.

The majority of male injection drug users in the United States have a steady relationship with a woman. The majority of these women partners are not injection drug users (Council on Scientific Affairs, 1989; Stone, Morisky, Detels, & Braxton, 1989; Raymond, 1988b; Mondanaro, 1987). Often the man's drug use is hidden from the partner out of fear of rejection or withdrawal of support. When condom use is initiated by the woman, it too has been reported to cause distrust, violence, and abandonment (Wermuth, Ham, & Robbins, 1991; Mays & Cochran, 1988). These reactions in ongoing relationships suggest precarious liaisons, in which the fear of losing a vital social bond discourages attempts to change sexual practices.

For women who either inject drugs or are involved with men who are addicted, the research points to additional dynamics that create barriers to reducing risks. Many of these women are in their childbearing years and restrict contraceptive use in order to get pregnant or because of perceived infertility (Wofsy, 1987; Ralph & Spigner, 1986). In addition, as already mentioned, these women may feel a lack of power in influencing the sexual expectations and preferences of their partners. Puerto Rican women interviewed in drug treatment programs in New York stated that they wanted their partners to use condoms, but felt unable to ask out of fear of being rejected (Worth & Rodriguez, 1987). They also feared deviating from the role expectation that they not discuss sex or birth control. As we discuss further below, conversations about condom use and the renegotiation of sexual practices are often even more difficult and threatening than discussions about drug use (Wermuth et al., 1991). Women who inject drugs with their male partners may be additionally vulnerable to HIV transmission through sharing of needles, with the man using the needle first. Rosenbaum's (1981a) study of sex roles among women heroin addicts found that women "assume a dependent role in the actual physical administration of the drug" (p. 863). A majority of the women in Rosenbaum's study had shared a needle with someone else; only 1/3 had ever injected heroin alone. By contrast, 3/4 of the men had injected heroin alone. "Hence those most intimate aspects of using heroin, which involve sharing the actual injection of the drug and the needle which is used, were practiced more by women than men" (p. 863).

As described in Chapter 5, the concept of self-efficacy has played an important role in researchers' attempts to understand what enables individuals to change risky sexual and drug use practices and to sustain those changes over time. When individuals believe they can exercise control over actions and situations that might pose a risk for HIV infection, they are more likely to exercise that control (Bandura, 1989). However, the extent to which this holds true for individuals with less actual control over their material and relational worlds remains to be learned. For example, Mondanaro (1987) points out that women at greatest risk for AIDS are those with the least amount of control over their lives. There may be real constraints on one's ability to maintain a self-efficacious cognitive state: "[D]enying [one's] vulnerability to AIDS or assuming the fatalistic attitude that she will contract the disease no matter what precautions she takes may be the woman's only defense" (Mondanaro, 1987, p. 146). A key factor in AIDS prevention among this group may be to bring about changes substantial enough to allow for a view of the disease as equal to or higher in importance than other dangers faced by women (Mays & Cochran, 1988). The extent of control over one's daily life also has implications for the practical aspects of HIV sexual prevention. Poor and addicted women are less likely to have ready access to condoms and spermicide, and the same will most likely be true for the "female condom" when it becomes available. Thus, in relationships, living conditions, and access to preventive supplies and helpful services, these women face the greatest obstacles in attempting to protect themselves.

This partial review of the literature suggests a need for preventive actions on several levels, from the grassroots up and from the outside inward to local milieux. Conduits for HIV prevention include the local and national print and broadcast media, the schools and local community agencies and churches, health care and drug treatment providers, and specially funded outreach and counseling programs. In addition, individual counseling that offers both education and help in problem solving with regard to HIV risk behaviors can have a profound impact on individuals' perceptions, intentions, and behaviors.

REACHING WOMEN SEXUAL PARTNERS OF DRUG-INJECTING MEN

To some extent, all of the avenues mentioned above are useful in reaching women and encouraging them to protect themselves from HIV. But diverse channels and forums are needed to reach the wide array of women at risk. In addition, women need more than messages; accessible services must accompany advice and information. Medical care, HIV antibody testing, counseling, and drug treatment are out of reach to many women without transportation or child care assistance. Here we describe a variety of avenues for reaching women at risk and their varied effectiveness in reaching different groups of women.

The Mass Media

Newspaper and radio coverage of the problem of sexual transmission and pediatric AIDS cases has been helpful in alerting women. Programmatic media efforts that have specifically targeted women sexual partners of drug injectors have been small-scale, such as video presentations or brochures. More widely broadcast messages have been aimed at gay men and heterosexuals, and have not adequately addressed the specific risk circumstances of women partners of drug injectors.

Women at risk for HIV are varied, and consequently, so are the methods needed to attract their attention. Newspaper ads may be the method most likely to tap working women with stable, busy lifestyles. Different newspapers will reach different subgroups within that category. Middle-class African-American women may be reached through a small newspaper with an African-American subscribership, while middle-class whites may be reached by other papers. Small, ethnic-group-oriented newspapers, sometimes neighborhood-based, may be the best way to speak to women within such groups—in their own languages and with a message in tune with their cultures. Thus, a variety of newspapers can be employed, of both large and small circulations, appealing to particular groups that may be geographically concentrated or spread out. Spanish-language radio programs may be the best medium for reaching unacculturated Hispanic women.

Medical Clinics

Health care providers have attempted to educate and counsel individual women about their possible risks for HIV infection. In addition, HIV antibody testing and counseling have been provided by private and public health facilities. Health care settings provide opportunities to reach a steady flow of women. Especially important are clinics offering obstetrical, gynecological, and pediatric care to large numbers of women. Clinical programs should be most aggressive in HIV prevention in areas with significant drug injection and cocaine use. Videos played and brochures displayed in waiting rooms allow women to become aware of and better educated about HIV risk. Intake screening can include questions about sexual partners, drug use, and sexual practices. Health providers can invite questions about AIDS and discuss possible risks with their patients. The medical setting potentially provides a private, professional, and nonjudgmental atmosphere in which individuals can be counseled without fear of reprisals. In addition, practitioners can provide referrals and liaison to other providers, easing the way for women who lack experience in utilizing services.

Drug Treatment Clinics

Drug treatment facilities and self-help programs can promote AIDS prevention in numerous ways, including making literature, speakers, and safe sex supplies available; providing individual and group counseling; and making referrals. Many drug treatment programs now offer HIV prevention counseling, HIV antibody testing, and referral to medical follow-up for infected individuals. Many counselors actively pursue the issue of AIDS risk in their counseling sessions, and some encourage clients to bring in their partners as well. Support groups for women, men, and couples can help alter norms in favor of safer sexual practices, and can foster mutual support and a sense of empowerment among peers. Chapter 6 provides a full discussion of HIV prevention and care in drug treatment programs.

AIDS Prevention Projects

Efforts to reach women at risk outside of clinical settings have been made in several cities, most often as an extension of efforts to reach injection drug users with preventive messages (Nova Research Company, 1990). Outreach programs, education campaigns, and phone lines can be enhanced to provide counseling and information to women concerned about AIDS risk. Media campaigns can increase awareness of such services by inviting women to call and ask questions. In addition, projects to address HIV risk in women can "piggyback" on existing outreach and research projects, to maximize the impact of existing services and resources.

Targeting Heterosexual Men

AIDS prevention to lower risk of sexual transmission must also target heterosexual men. An array of male role models (e.g., sports stars, respected officials, community leaders) can present positive messages regarding protecting loved ones as well as oneself, and can encourage the proper use of condoms. Men can also be encouraged to communicate with their women partners in the same way that women are being encouraged to discuss the issue with their male partners. In this way, messages and prevention campaigns can encourage men and women to share the task of initiating discussion and reaching agreements about mutual protection from HIV infection.

A PROJECT TO COUNSEL WOMEN AT RISK

Here we provide a model of individual AIDS prevention counseling tailored to women who may be at risk for HIV infection in their sexual relationships with men. It is designed to be added to the routines of health care providers, drug treatment counselors, outreach workers, and therapists. Even if women are knowledgeable about AIDS, they can benefit from discussion of their individual circumstances. A private, one-on-one counseling session provides the opportunity to ask questions specific to a woman's situation, or questions she is embarrassed to ask with others present.

The counseling model described below was developed for a study of women sexual partners of injection drug users in the San Francisco Bay Area, called the Partners Outreach Project. Women were recruited through injection drug users entering treatment, through chain referral, through newspaper ads, and through fliers distributed to clinics and posted in high-risk neighborhoods. Seventy-seven women were enrolled in the study. They were randomly assigned to either a control condition of one informational session of AIDS prevention counseling, or an experimental condition of three sessions of problem-solving counseling in addition to information. Baseline and follow-up interviews included questions about AIDS knowledge, birth control, sexual practices, partners' needle use practices, HIV testing history of self and partner, and questions about relationships. Open-ended questions probed each woman's thoughts about her HIV risk and her relationships. The responses (which are described below) often revealed strategies by which women attempted to reduce their risk.

The Partners Outreach Project reached a diverse group of women sexual partners. However, the respondents were most likely skewed toward a group with higher education and more stable living conditions than the general population of women sexual partners of injection drug users in the United States. The average age of women in the study was 33 years, ranging from 19 to 57 years. Of the 77 women, 40 were white, 28 were African-American, 7 were Hispanic, and 1 was Native American. Fifty-four had at least a high school education. The majority (45) were either married or living with their sexual partners. Sixty-one had children. Twenty-five of the women were employed full- or part-time, and 30 received some kind of public assistance (Aid to Families with Dependent Children, General Assistance, and/or Social Security Insurance). These women were generally knowledgeable about AIDS. Nearly half had themselves used injection drugs at some time since 1978. (Women who had injected drugs in the past 6 months were screened out.) The majority of the women's sexual partners had injected drugs during the past year (58); 28 were shooting daily; and about half of the partners had shared needles during the past year. The women had averaged three sexual partners during the prior year, and 46 reported never using condoms in the history of their current relationships.

Partners Counseling Protocol

The following guidelines provide a framework for counselors and health care practitioners to counsel their women patients or clients regarding HIV prevention. The protocol was designed for three 1-hour-long sessions of counseling, but it can be abbreviated or extended, depending upon the number of contacts and the amount of time available.

ASKING ABOUT A WOMAN'S CONCERNS AND CIRCUMSTANCES

Practitioners need not be afraid to ask women whether they have concerns about AIDS. Questions can be added to routine screening forms: Does she have sex with a man who injects drugs? Does she inject drugs herself? Does she trade sex for drugs or money? Does she have plans for pregnancy? If the professional is at ease and asks these questions with sensitivity, many women will welcome the opportunity to discuss their concerns privately. Women's statements often reveal information about risk behaviors and about their ability to acknowledge that risk. A woman's descriptions also may provide information about her relationships and living conditions. These are issues that must be addressed if the practitioner is to suggest changes credibly.

INFORMING HER ABOUT HIV AND WAYS TO PROTECT AGAINST INFECTION

In stating her concerns, the woman may ask questions about AIDS, such as "If my partner is infected, could I catch it from him by kissing?" Her statements may also reveal misconceptions, such as "My partner is very clean with his 'works' [drug-injecting supplies], so I'm not too worried about AIDS." Statements such as these help set the agenda for the educational part of the counseling, which is most effective when it takes its cues from the woman's statements. Education also involves a discussion of modes of transmission and precautions that can be taken in sexual behavior and drug use behavior. A counselor should relax and discuss these issues comfortably, not worrying about including every important fact during the discussion. In wrapping up, the counselor refers to a counseling checklist of important points (see Table 9.1) and gives the sheet of information to the woman to take with her. This format maximizes attention to the woman's personal concerns and helps to maintain a comfortable conversation, while also providing her with thorough information. Whenever possible, written materials should be in the native languages of those counseled.

TABLE 9.1. Counseling Women about HIV Risk: A Checklist

Ask:	What are her concerns? Does she inject drugs? Does a partner inject drugs? Does she use birth control? Is she pregnant? Planning pregnancy? What are her thoughts about condoms? What are her partner's thoughts about condoms? Have they discussed condom use?
Inform her:	About routes of transmission About methods of prevention About condoms and nonoxynol-9 About the role of HIV antibody testing About birth control and pregnancy
Practice:	With condoms With spermicidal creams, jellies, foams Bringing up the subject with a partner Responding to reactions from a partner
Emphasize:	She can call you back HIV infection can be prevented Identify her supports Encourage her to take care of herself

PROBLEM SOLVING IN REGARD TO SITUATIONS OF RISK

Once it is clear which situations, relationships, and behaviors are putting the woman at risk, the counselor asks how any of these might be changed. What could the woman do to reduce her risk? The counselor presses the woman to consider whether these are realistic goals; if so, the woman generates a list of steps by which she could bring them about. It is up to the counselor to set the woman at ease by being nonjudgmental, giving her time to think, and reminding her that only she can make these decisions. The woman is encouraged to devise a prevention plan—for example, to use condoms with her partner, to get HIV antibody testing (and to encourage her partner to do so), and to request a commitment from her partner not to engage in risky behaviors. The counseling provides the woman with the opportunity to think ahead to how she will handle situations and relationships in which partners may refuse to cooperate with a plan to avoid risk.

IDENTIFYING SOURCES OF SUPPORT

Needs for support may be material, emotional, or social, and can be addressed in order of the most immediate concern to the woman. The counselor helps by identifying and writing down names and phone numbers of people and services that may be helpful. Liaison with other agencies can be helpful—a phone call to another provider can smooth the way for the woman to get her needs met. Encouragement also helps women take steps toward accomplishing their plan to avoid HIV infection. Up-to-date referrals are needed, and access to a telephone can greatly help. Bus tokens can make it possible for a woman and her children to get to and from appointments, and inexpensive child care services can greatly ease the burden of women in high-risk living conditions. Unfortunately, these services remain scarce despite the pervasive need. At the close of counseling, the counselor invites the woman to call if she has more questions, needs referrals, or wishes to talk further about her situation.

WOMEN'S STRATEGIES AND CLINICAL ISSUES

Uncertainty is the first problem women face when they realize their risk for AIDS through sex. A woman often cannot be sure that her partner has used only new or cleaned needles and that he is free of HIV infection. How do women cope with this lack of assurance about such a grave risk? They do so in a variety of ways. Often they reduce or eliminate their own injection drug use and enter drug treatment (Wermuth et al., 1991). If not already monogamous, they often reduce their number of sexual partners and pay more attention to their partners' other sexual relationships. Condom use may not be the first or preferred method to protect against HIV, but it is often considered by women who know they are at risk in their sexual relationships. Described below are five categories of coping strategies that emerged from analysis of baseline questionnaire items, including taped responses to open-ended items. The strategies described are as follows: talking with partners; sizing up the costs and benefits of pressing for condom use; getting tested for the HIV antibody; influencing partners' needle use practices; and making changes in relationships. We also discuss anxiety and denial of risk as the emotional effects of imperfect strategies to guard against HIV infection.

Talking with Partners

Although some couples in which one partner is an injection drug user avoid the topic of AIDS, others talk about their risk and discuss (or argue about) the idea of using condoms. Agreements to use condoms do not necessarily result from these negotiations, however. And although possessing "communication skills" may help in one's efforts to persuade, they do not guarantee a partner's agreement to use condoms. The subject raises sensitive issues of loyalty, trust, and sexual performance, and may evoke disputes that threaten relationships. Proposals to use condoms sometimes provoke accusations and counteraccusations. In addition, condoms can loom as a threat to the man's control over the couple's sexual relationship, and, because of the mechanics of condom use, can raise fears about sexual performance. Especially for couples who have never used condoms, their barrier nature may take on a larger, symbolic importance (as in "I need to protect myself from you with this").

A majority of sexually active women may be willing to have their partners use condoms if they perceive themselves to be at risk for HIV. In one study, among 756 women attending contraceptive care clinics, a majority endorsed condom use to prevent HIV. Statistical predictors of condom use in this study were acceptance of condom advertisement, perceived male and peer acceptance of condoms, and the effect of condom use on the enjoyment of sexual intercourse (Valdiserri, Arena, Proctor, & Bonati, 1989). Half of the women in the Partners Outreach Project had either talked about condoms or used them with a partner in the past month. And content analysis of qualitative transcripts revealed that some women who suggested condom use were accused of having AIDS by their male partners (9 of 77).

Sizing Up the Costs and Benefits

Women size up the costs and benefits of pressing their partners to use condoms in much the same way they size up the costs and benefits of taking contraceptive risks (Luker, 1975). Factors that may influence their thoughts and feelings include partners' attitudes and anticipated reactions, reluctance to provoke major breaches in relationships, and the women's own ambivalence about pressing for condom use. The issue of condom use and the proposal to alter sexual routines may threaten major disruptions, which both members of a couple may want to avoid. Moreover, some women themselves are ambivalent about or reject the idea of regular condom use. These several factors mitigate against women's pressing their partners to the point of giving ultimatums.

When first interviewed in the Partners Outreach Project, 15 of 77 women had already experienced negative reactions from their partners regarding using condoms. An additional 22 women anticipated negative reactions should they raise the subject. Content analysis of responses to open-ended questions revealed higher levels of angry responses, with 33 (43%) of women reporting negative responses by their partners. Examples included a man's verbally accosting or physically assaulting a woman or accusing her of having AIDS, being unfaithful, or being crazy.

HIV Antibody Testing

Women sexual partners of injection drug users who are concerned about AIDS may seek out testing for themselves and encourage their partners to get tested as well. Receiving negative test results can provide at least temporary relief from worry and boost motivation to avoid becoming infected in the future. For others, however, testing provides reassurance of avoided infection without a resolution to maintain safe practices. In such cases, negative test results fuel rationalizations (e.g., "If I'm not infected now after what I've done, I'm not going to get infected"). For some women in our project, the issue of testing was more complicated. Often testing raised feelings of ambivalence about acknowledging risk and issues of trust and loyalty in their relationships. Such was the case for Katherine, whose partner shared needles and refused to use condoms. (We have substituted fictitious names in our case examples.) She intended to be tested but had delayed doing it:

> *"I would like to take the test to see if I am [infected], but personally I don't think that I have it. I don't use drugs intravenously, I have only had one sex partner within the last 4 years, so if I do have it, it's from him."*

Negative HIV antibody test results may reinforce a system of denial, providing a rationalization for not using condoms. A man who has injected drugs and who reports a negative HIV antibody test result to his partner may use this as "proof" to her that she is not going to get infected and that condom use is not needed. Thus, partners who get tested for the HIV antibody and receive negative test results do not necessarily have cooperative attitudes about using condoms to prevent future infection (Wermuth, Ham, & Hester, 1989). Women may then feel defensive and be hard put to argue for condom use without specific evidence that their partners are engaging in risky needle use or sexual practices. Moreover, women do not have access to their partners' test results and cannot verify whether they are being told the truth. Men who fear loss of their relationships if infected may lie about positive results in order not to lose their partners. Women who are reassured by their own negative test results are still dependent upon their partners' cooperation in preventing sexual transmission of HIV.

Couples in which both know of the man's HIV infection may behave quite differently from those in which infection status is unknown. Perhaps willingness to report a positive result to a partner entails a level of trust that the relationship will not be lost as a result. Also, the shared knowledge of infection may motivate both the man and the woman to avoid sexual transmission cooperatively, whether by agreeing to use condoms, by engaging in sexual practices other than intercourse, or by avoiding sex altogether.

Despite the trauma of learning of a positive antibody test result—or perhaps because of it—the news can move couples to be safer in their sexual practices. However, there certainly are some individuals who know but do not tell their partners that they are HIV-infected. Still others avoid testing because they fear a positive result. In addition, women may choose not to report slips in their "consistent" condom use to interviewers or counselors. In one case a woman with an infected husband had a baby during the course of the study, although in baseline and follow-up interviews she reported always using condoms.

At entry to the Partners Outreach Project, 61% of the women had already been tested for HIV antibodies, and they reported that 51% of their partners also had been tested. An additional 13% of the women did not know whether their partners had been tested. Two women reported receiving positive HIV antibody test results, and eight reported that their male partners had received positive test results. Statistically significant predictors of a woman's having received HIV antibody testing were the woman's having a past history of injection drug use, participation in a methadone maintenance program, and known HIV infection in sexual partner (Wermuth, Falcone, & Sorensen, 1990b). All couples with a known infected member reported practicing safer sex (seven) or abstinence (one). Infrequent sex also seemed to be an adjustment these couples made: Seven of the nine couples with an infected individual reported no sex (oral, anal, or vaginal) during the past 30 days.

Influencing Partners' Needle Use Practices

Many women perceive their AIDS risk in terms of the drug use behavior of their partners. If only their partners would stop injecting drugs, or clean their needles, or never share with others, they would be free from risk. For example, Georgia stated:

> *"My husband and I have discussed [AIDS risk] and now he doesn't share his needles, he cleans them out. . . . I keep an eye on him and watch what he does so he doesn't infect me."*

Testing is often combined with an attempt to improve the safety of partners' needle practices, providing reassurance that the couple has not yet been infected and that current practices will not result in infection.

The inconvenient aspects of condoms are not the only reason for their lack of popularity among couples with an injection drug user. For most couples, negotiations about drug use practices are less threatening than negotiations about condom use. Couples have histories of discussing drug use, and however conflictual that topic, negotiations over sex are likely to be far more volatile. Proposed changes in drug use can be couched in terms of protecting the man as well as the woman and do not necessarily disrupt existing sexual routines or power dynamics. By contrast, a woman's proposal that her partner use condoms can raise issues of trust and loyalty, anxieties about sexual performance, and issues of power and control. Especially in couples new to condom use, the introduction of the barrier method can symbolize distancing and distrust.

In the course of answering open-ended questions in the Partners Outreach Project, without being specifically asked about methods they had used to influence partners, 23% of the subjects reported attempts to persuade their partners to alter drug use practices as a way to protect themselves against AIDS. Examples included cleaning partners' needles; finding supplies of sterile needles; educating partners about risk from needle sharing; and convincing the partners to inject drugs only at home, alone, or with select individuals. These attempts to "domesticate" partners' drug use allowed for greater surveillance of their partners' practices. Limiting drug-using associates and keeping drug use at home most likely reduced AIDS risk for the men, and in turn for the women as well. In one case, Eleanor persuaded her husband to inject drugs only at home, but she still worried about what he would do when he was with his friends:

> *"I was so worried about this. . . . that I put the [small bleach] bottles in the glove compartment of the car, thinking if [he shot up he might] have enough sense to run outside and get the bottle of bleach. . . . [I tell him,] 'even though you have your own needle, take the bleach because there is always somebody who doesn't have a needle, and they are going to want to use yours.'"*

Changes in Relationships

There are important differences in negotiating about HIV risk in casual versus long-term relationships. The possibility of painful and violent confrontations is present in both, but in long-term relationships the ramifications are of far greater consequence. Women who are in marital or quasi-marital relationships with men who inject drugs, and who are economically or emotionally dependent upon these men, may not want to threaten the loss of their relationships. Also, when a couple shares children the woman may not want to lose the children's contact with the father, or she may wish to preserve the semblance of an "intact" family.

The changes women make to protect themselves from HIV infection in long-term relationships often fit into existing caretaking roles. Adding AIDS concerns and precautions in the area of drug use to that role is most often less problematic than confronting partners with pressure to use condoms. As mentioned above, such confrontations can threaten fragile arrangements and provoke angry responses and accusations. However, it may also be the case that women who have shared the ups and downs of their partners' heroin (or cocaine) habit may be sufficiently discontent to end relationships (Rosenbaum, 1981b), and AIDS risk may provide the final impetus for their exit.

Examples of changes in relationships that reduce risk of HIV infection for the woman without forcing the issue of condom use include having sex less often, having sex with fewer sexual partners, and separating from partners. Avoidance of sex may be a strategy being used widely by women with partners thought to pose an AIDS risk. As a woman who had seen her partner share needles reported,

> *"That's the reason why we haven't had sex for the past month, because I know what he thinks about the condom and everything. . . . we've been together 7 years and he's never had one on."*

Baseline data suggested that avoiding sex was an HIV prevention strategy for several of the women. Twenty-one of the women reported in open-ended interviews having no sexual intercourse during the past 30 days, and an additional 49 reported having only one sexual partner in the past 30 days. This information, combined with the mention of being more careful about whom they were having sex with, suggests that for at least some women reducing sexual contacts was part of their strategy to lower their risk. However, we cannot be certain of the extent of the change, since we do not have information about the prior frequency of sex.

Emotional Effects of Imperfect Strategies: Denial and Anxiety

Women downplay or deny their risk for AIDS to varying degrees. Denial of risk sometimes involves holding contradictory thoughts about their risk—for example, acknowledging risk in one part of a discussion or interview, and denying it in another. Denial can also be manifested in a woman's inability to acknowledge the fact that she is at risk in her sexual relationship. She may be articulate and animated about her partner's AIDS risk, but draw a blank when asked to describe her own risk. In an extreme case, flattened affect suggested a woman's emotional blockage of the whole problem. She calmly related that her husband shared needles regularly, that they never used condoms, and that she realized she could get AIDS this way. Unlike the majority of other women in the study who were eager to talk about their circumstances and ask questions in private, this individual showed no outward signs of worry and had little interest in talking about her situation. This woman's depression seemed partly the cause and partly the result of the several other problems she had in addition to her risk for HIV, including her own drug abuse, lack of decision-making power in her relationships, and responsibility for the care of their two children.

Women often remain anxious about their HIV risk despite substantial efforts to reduce uncertainty and gain greater control. In the Partners Outreach Project, women in long-term relationships often wanted to trust their men and to believe they cared enough to protect them from AIDS. The following remarks by a woman in the study reveal her mix of vigilance, trust, and anxiety. When asked what she could do to keep herself from getting AIDS, Georgia described what she was already doing:

"I am sure that he doesn't mess around with other women, so I am not concerned about that. It's only the needles. I have no choice but to trust him enough to think about me and his son."

Strategies of getting HIV antibody testing plus attempts to influence partners' needle practices in the direction of greater safety are often preferred to pressuring men to use condoms. As noted earlier, many couples have vocabularies and repertoires for discussing drug use and established roles for coping with that problem. Proposed changes in drug use can be couched in terms of protecting the man as well as the woman, whereas the same can be said for discussions about condoms only when both partners have positive attitudes about their use.

The strategy to influence partners' drug use practices toward safety is consistent with the caretaking role of many women in relationships with men who inject drugs. The interpretation often given to such behavior is that it is "enabling" their men partners' drug use and a function of their "codependent relationships." Although many relationships between men drug users and their women partners are relatively rigid and emotionally "enmeshed," it is also the case that many individuals in these relationships develop rational strategies and make rational choices in efforts to prevent HIV infection. Exercising influence over a man's drug use in the direction of safety may fit into a caretaker role, but the motivations may be rational and the consequences positive. In other words, it is overly simplistic to interpret all actions by women partners of drug-injecting men through the lens of dependency on drug users. Instead, attitudes and behaviors need to be weighed in light of the circumstances of women in these relationships and the real outcomes of the strategies they pursue.

ADVANTAGES AND LIMITATIONS OF INDIVIDUAL COUNSELING

Individual counseling does not hold the only key to prevention, but among its advantages is the fact that women can address their own personal and circumstantial issues privately with a counselor. If self-efficacy is a key psychological variable in being able to take steps to protect oneself, then individual counseling may operate as a catalyst in bringing about this frame of mind. The most powerful aspect of individual counseling is the opportunity for a woman to focus on her personal risk for an HIV infection in a private discussion with a knowledgeable and caring individual. This allows the woman to ask questions she might not address with others and to examine the risks she may be taking. The support given by the counselor may help to empower the woman to protect herself.

Peer counseling can be especially effective in establishing trust and addressing the conditions that impede women's efforts to protect themselves. The National AIDS Demonstration Research (NADR) Project, funded by the National Institute on Drug Abuse, was based on a peer outreach model. The NADR curriculum for prevention education and counseling was based on the principles of meeting women where they are, empowering them, and learning from them (Nova Research Company, 1990). The San Francisco project site included the use of a "storefront" location (a "room of one's own") where women could come in, relax, talk, and find out about resources and services.

Ideally, individual counseling is combined with numerous other preventive efforts, including those in the mass media, schools, medical and drug abuse clinics and hospitals, and community and grassroots endeavors. Individual counseling usually does not involve sexual partners, although this could have a powerful impact if added as a second stage of counseling. In addition, individual counseling does not directly affect group norms or foster group support for individuals' efforts. Nor does it affect the level of institutional supports available to individuals in danger of HIV infection. Because it is private and individualized, the impact on friends, family, and community is minimal and slow to evolve. In addition, it is impractical as a general approach because of the large numbers of individuals and the amount of labor that would be needed to reach and provide all with counseling. Programs that are public and group-oriented are therefore necessary adjuncts to individual and group clinical approaches. Finally, for those women at highest risk, individual AIDS prevention counseling does not have the potential to provide solutions to problems of violence, addiction, and poverty in their daily living conditions, and therefore may have only limited impact (Worth, 1989).

SUMMARY

Women do not assess their AIDS risk only in terms of their sexual contacts or their own drug injecting. Rather, women take into account what they perceive as the source of their risk—their male partners' drug injecting. Additional uncertainties make assessments of risk problematic for this group. Most importantly, these include lack of complete knowledge about their male partners' needle use practices, possible homosexual practices, and HIV antibody test results. Yet, even when knowledgeable about partners' needle sharing and the possibility of transmission through sex, many women deny or downplay their risk of becoming infected. This is often frustrating to the AIDS prevention counselor, but should not be surprising; people generally tend not to believe that they will be victims of negative life events, including serious illness (Weinstein, 1980, 1982). If solutions seem out of reach, anxiety may cause individuals to block out the reality of their risk.

Many women and their partners reduce their HIV risk in ways that do not involve the use of condoms—for example, by combining HIV antibody testing with safer needle practices. In some cases, men's drug use becomes "domesticated," with the men agreeing to inject drugs only at home, alone, or only with selected individuals. These and other strategies reduce HIV risk, though most often they do not eliminate it. Overall, the remedies adopted by women as described above reveal preferences by the men—and often by women as well—to avoid the use of condoms. Couples tend to avoid negotiations about their sexual relationships, thereby sidestepping sensitive issues of loyalty, sexual performance, and control.

Addicted, poor, and socially marginal women may be less inclined to register their AIDS risk consciously, and may also be less able to avoid risky situations and behaviors. The association between poverty and mental health problems is well documented (Belle, 1990), and the increasing numbers of women with children living in poverty have implications for HIV risk. Nonetheless, certain factors may increase the likelihood that women will acknowledge their HIV risk. For example, we found that women whose partners were currently injecting drugs were nearly three times as likely to perceive themselves at risk (Wermuth et al., 1990a). From an AIDS prevention point of view, it is encouraging that women's perceptions of risk are in part based upon the actual behaviors (i.e., partners' drug injection) that result in women's risk in sex. To avoid risk, women sexual partners of injection drug users are dependent upon their partners' cessation of risky needle practices and their willingness to use condoms. Lack of female-controlled methods of HIV prevention underlies and exacerbates these difficulties (Stein, 1990). Incomplete knowledge about their partners' practices and lack of control over condom use put women—especially those in long-term relationships—in a bind.

Since relationships are the contexts in which negotiations about sexual practices occur (or fear and avoidance of those negotiations), they should be included among the variables we study. Models of health-related behaviors based upon individualistic conceptions of risk may be inadequate to address the problem of the sexual transmission of HIV. In addition, the public health recommendation that individuals have just one sexual partner to avoid AIDS risk may cause confusion among couples with a drug injector. A monogamous relationship with a man who has a history of injection drug use does not provide safety from HIV risk. Moreover, solutions to risk require open and honest communication, and proposing condom use often evokes distrust, especially in marital or "steady" relationships.

As noted earlier, programmatic media efforts specifically targeted to women sexual partners of injection drug users have been small-scale, such as video presentations or brochures. More widely broadcast media messages have been aimed at heterosexuals generally, and do not speak to the circumstances of women partners of injection drug users. For example, monogamy is not a solution to this group's risk. The variations among women and their partners are also important. Cultural and socioeconomic differences call for varied approaches. Moreover, messages about condom use often presume that both members of the couple have an equal ability to implement their use, when this is most likely not the case. Women are dependent on the active cooperation of their male partners in preventing sexual transmission of HIV, whether it be through HIV antibody testing, changes in drug use habits, or consistent and effective use of condoms.

Part 3

SOCIAL IMPLICATIONS

Chapter 10

Adopting Effective Interventions

JAMES L. SORENSEN
JOSEPH R. GUYDISH

If nobody knows about a great technique for preventing AIDS, then it will not have a wide impact. This chapter is about the application of knowledge and techniques: how to move useful prevention projects from the developmental stages into the field. The chapter is aimed at two groups. A primary audience consists of the many professionals who must decide what prevention programs should be adopted in their health care setting. The coordinator of a county's drug abuse programs, for example, wants to sponsor AIDS prevention efforts that fit best with the county's population and budget. The developers of interventions comprise a second audience. For them, the question is how to get their interventions out into the field.

The chapter first considers the problem from the point of view of "adopters"—the people selecting AIDS prevention techniques for their local use. The chapter suggests that people considering an intervention base their selection on understanding why people do risky things, assess the evidence that an intervention is effective, and build their own evaluation into their adoption plans. The chapter also points to critical gaps in prevention research, warning adopters that there are many limitations to the existing prevention studies.

The next part of the chapter has suggestions for "disseminators"—the developers of interventions or the people who want to see that effective interventions get into the field. It reviews lessons from the dissemination literature: namely, that the effective interventions are not always adopted; that research that compares dissemination methods exists; and that one lesson is the importance of personal contact. We conclude the chapter with several recommendations for the adoption and dissemination of effective AIDS prevention programs.

Before going further, we want to explain about one of our attempts at AIDS prevention that did not work. The story illustrates the importance of developing preventive interventions wisely.

In spring 1985, our San Francisco General Hospital (SFGH) Outpatient Detoxification Clinic was looking for ways to reduce AIDS risks in the heroin abusers who came into treatment. At the same time, the San Francisco AIDS Foundation launched San Francisco's first AIDS awareness campaign for drug abusers. It included a billboard reading "DON'T SHARE," with an 8-foot-long syringe. The clinic obtained a spare billboard from the AIDS Foundation to mount on a wall in the clinic waiting room. For the months of March and April, we had been asking drug abusers at intake into the program how many times they were sharing needles, and with how many people. On April 30 we put up the billboard, and we continued to ask. Some patients liked the billboard because it reminded them about AIDS. Others disliked it, saying it made them want to "fix." Staff members liked the billboard because it communicated AIDS awareness and brightened up the wall. The proportion of applicants who reported needle sharing was 57% in March, 52% in April (before the billboard went up), 49% in May (right after the billboard went up), but back up to 57% in June. We concluded that the billboard was useful clinically, but that it was not sufficient to decrease even drug users' self-reports of needle sharing, much less their actual risk behaviors. It had some small "shock value," but patients quickly became immune to it.

SUGGESTIONS FOR ADOPTING EFFECTIVE INTERVENTIONS

A public health planner who wants to prevent AIDS with drug users and their sexual partners is faced with a dizzying array of options. Interventions might include increasing the availability of drug abuse treatment; promoting awareness with a media blitz; sponsoring workshops for health care workers; sponsoring a needle exchange; organizing street outreach by peer counselors; sponsoring the distribution of bleach, condoms, or dental dams; targeting at-risk youths for prevention messages; conducting outreach to sex industry workers; working with pediatric and prenatal clinics to educate women about AIDS; sponsoring a crackdown on illicit drug use; sponsoring HIV antibody testing and counseling programs; changing laws to liberalize the availability of sterile syringes; conducting contact tracing of AIDS or HIV-infected cases; or reaching participants at clinics treating sexually transmitted diseases. These are a few of the dozens of approaches that have been attempted.

Every approach has its advocates, and few health care systems can do all of them. Those advocating each approach may claim that it is effective, exciting, or at least feasible in the local setting. The people responsible for choosing approaches may not be experts themselves. How can a planner decide which ones are best for the particular setting? Public health professionals, because of their specialized training in disease prevention and health promotion, may provide helpful consultation when deciding which programs to adopt. We have several suggestions that can help a potential adopter in the process of selecting interventions to prevent the spread of AIDS with drug users or their sexual partners (see Table 10.1).

Basing the Intervention on Understanding

One principle is to learn why drug users or sexual partners engage in the behaviors that put them at risk. The reasons may include ignorance of transmission routes; lack of supplies that would promote safe needle use or safe sex; lack of intent to take care of themselves and disregard of risks to the people they might infect with HIV; or embarrassment about taking precautions. No intervention will be right for all of these reasons, but some will be better than others.

The advantage of the the billboard approach described above was that it alerted drug users to the AIDS–drug connection. However, the billboard did little to change their motivation: It merely told them what *not* to do.

Ethnographic research methods have made a contribution to understanding the motivations for taking AIDS risks. Ethnographers have established rapport and trust with the subjects of their studies and have been able to observe incidents in natural settings. These methods have yielded valuable information on the meaning and practices of sharing needles (Des Jarlais, Friedman, & Strug, 1986) and behavior

TABLE 10.1. Suggestions for Adopting AIDS Prevention Techniques

1. Understand the people who need to be reached
   - Ethnographic investigations
   - Informal consultations
2. Assess the evidence of effectiveness
   - Published studies
   - Participant opinions
3. Evaluate local effectiveness (include evaluation in the intervention plan)

patterns in shooting galleries (Page, Chitwood, Smith, Kane, & McBride, 1990; Watters, 1989). In some communities, health planners may benefit by sponsoring ethnographic work initially to clarify the local patterns, locations, and motivations for risk behaviors. Another way to learn more about the target of interventions is to invite them in for consultations about possible intervention techniques; such consultations may include brainstorming sessions or focus groups.

Assessing Evidence That Interventions Work

Potential adopters of interventions can select from the menu of intervention options in the same way they wisely purchase any item or service. They can examine the written research on the intervention, giving more credibility to independently conducted evaluations. They can talk with former participants in the intervention, or contact experts for their opinions. It should be kept in mind that an intervention may be effective in one cultural group and ineffective in another; nevertheless, some evidence of efficacy is better than none. The National Academy of Sciences has recently published an expanded guide to evaluating AIDS prevention programs, which can provide criteria on which to judge contending interventions (Coyle, Boruch, & Turner, 1990). A recent article by Lorion (1990) reviews 10 lessons from psychotherapy research that apply to evaluating AIDS prevention programs. The Appendix to this book lists a number of organizations that may have expert consultants who can help in the selection process.

Evaluating How Well the Intervention Works in a Particular Setting

The decision to adopt a program is the beginning rather than the end of an evaluation. To judge how well an intervention works in a particular setting, the adopter will specify goals in advance of implementing the project, selecting objectives for the program that are measurable. An evaluation plan ought to go with an intervention, in order to document how well it accomplished the goals that were set out for it. One focus may be on "process" objectives (i.e., measures of how well the process of the intervention is mounted). These include such measures as meeting the timetable for project management and attendance by target participants. Another form of evaluation is accounting for services provided by the program, such as number of persons counseled or number of presentations made in a specified period of time. Records describing the client population served can later be used to refocus prevention efforts at groups that have been missed. In most interventions it will also be feasible to collect simple outcome measures, such as participants' satisfaction with the intervention.

We realize that people adopting interventions are not necessarily experts in evaluation. It may be important for such people to attend meetings where the evaluations of interventions are presented, to contact social scientists on their community board or in local universities, or to get help from organizations that are involved in the evaluation of public health interventions (see the Appendix).

The Main Points

The people with responsibility to adopt AIDS prevention programs have a difficult role. To be effective, they can start with the target population, aiming to learn as much as possible about why this population continues to be at risk. This kind of needs assessment has been helped by recent developments in ethnographic research, which is an excellent way of understanding the lives of participants who are at risk. Program adopters can also evaluate the existing evidence, to determine the relative efficacy of various types of programs in accomplishing the goal of preventing AIDS. Finally, no one can expect that an intervention can be taken "off the shelf" and be effective. It is important to evaluate how well it works in the local community. Planners must conduct evaluations in order to know whether the interventions they have selected are accomplishing their goals.

LIMITATIONS IN THE EVALUATION OF INTERVENTIONS

A person who is evaluating interventions for adoption and implementation should be aware of the weaknesses in the available research. Injection-drug-using populations are notoriously difficult to access and to follow over time. The interplay between them and the larger society is partially defined by the illegal nature of drug use and other activities through which users gain money and drugs. Consequently, this population exists within a loosely knit subculture with minimal ties to the larger society, to health care and public health personnel, and to academic communities. Drug users often adopt transient lifestyles, to elude detection by the law and to evade drug-related problems with others within the subculture. Transience may involve travel between cities, but more commonly involves frequent moves within a locale and the absence of a permanent home. Three significant methodological issues derive from the transient nature of injection-drug-using populations: reliance on in-treatment samples, cross-sectional designs, and self-report.

Reliance on In-Treatment Samples

Most available studies of seroprevalence rely on information collected from drug users in drug treatment programs. Des Jarlais et al. (1989a) attempted to generalize seroprevalence findings to out-of-treatment samples by restricting their sample to recent admissions, reasoning that these participants would have recent drug use patterns closely approximating those of people not in treatment. This strategy, although it approaches the methodological problem, is probably inadequate to allow generalization of results to the out-of-treatment population. Of 97 respondents not in treatment in one study, 53% reported that they would not enter treatment if it were immediately available (Watters, 1987). In a sample of HIV-affected drug users, half of whom were injectors, 46% reported that they were not interested in drug abuse treatment (Guydish, Temoshok, Dilley, & Rinaldi, 1990a). Although the proportion of injection drug users who do not contact treatment programs is not known, it is probably very large. Samples of in-treatment drug abusers may differ in important ways from the less accessible out-of-treatment drug users; these differences may include dimensions of seroprevalence, risk behavior, and degree to which their use of drugs is problematic.

With respect to evaluation of risk behavior, Selwyn included a sample of injectors in a narcotic detoxification unit of a detention facility, reasoning that these involuntarily incarcerated drug users might also differ from those not incarcerated (Selwyn, Feiner, Cox, Lipschutz, & Cohen, 1987). In the San Francisco studies of risk behavior, one small ethnographic study included out-of-treatment drug users (Watters, 1988), as did a study of needle cleaning (Watters, 1987) and a study of needle exchange (Clark et al., 1989). These reports, however, did not address differences between in-treatment and out-of-treatment injection drug users.

Reliance on Cross-Sectional Designs

The second methodological issue deriving from the transient nature of the population is the reliance on cross-sectional studies, with the concomitant absence of longitudinal data. Inferences regarding changes in seroprevalence and risk behavior over time are best based on longitudinal prospective cohort studies. Although such studies have been conducted with gay male populations (Winkelstein et al., 1988), there are no comparable longitudinal cohorts of injection drug users. This may be partially due to historically lower funding of drug abuse research or to the lack of longitudinal designs employed by addiction researchers; it is certainly due in part to significant problems encountered in finding and following this population. Several researchers have addressed this problem through repeated cross-sectional designs (Chaisson, Moss, Onishi, Osmond, & Carlson, 1987a; Chaisson, Osmond, Moss, Feldman, & Biernacki, 1987b; Chaisson et al., 1989), or through a "passive recapture" process, which culls out subjects who happen to participate in more than one cross-sectional sampling frame (Moss et al., 1989; Guydish, Abramowitz, Woods, Black, & Sorensen, 1990a). These strategies are limited by the initial sampling plan, however, which most often includes only people in drug abuse treatment. Recaptured in-treatment drug abuser samples do give some information regarding changes over time, but again give no information regarding out-of-treatment samples. Consequently, the ability to draw conclusions regarding changes in seroprevalence and risk behavior change over time is greatly hampered by the limited data available for out-of-treatment samples and by the absence of longitudinal studies.

Reliance on Self-Report

A third significant methodological weakness, specific to data concerning risk behavior change, is the almost complete reliance on self-report data. Needle sharing, needle cleaning, and sexual risk behavior, especially when linked to life-threatening disease, may be regarded as intimate and personal. This type of information, although necessary to enable appropriate public health interventions, may be awkward for participants to report and therefore difficult to access. Some studies have found self-reports of drug users to be accurate (Amsel, Mandell, Matthias, Mason, & Hocherman, 1976); however, respondents in such studies may be influenced by issues of social desirability, of confiding accurate risk behavior to researchers who may be affiliated with treatment programs, and of access to treatment. Consequently, the magnitude of risk behavior is likely to be heavily and frequently underreported.

Two strategies could be adopted in attempting to deal with self-report bias. One would involve validating self-report through measures using technological means—for example, testing needles collected from injection drug users with forensic tests designed to detect the presence of more than one blood type. Another strategy would be the development of non-self-report measures of risk behavior. Chitwood et al. (1990a), for example, recently tested needles collected from shooting galleries in Miami for the presence of HIV antibodies. Identifying and recapturing needles distributed by exchange programs would be a measure that similarly would not rely on self-report. Analogously, it may be possible to test any sample of needles for the presence of HIV antibodies. Although such methodologies are not yet in use, their successful development and application would significantly enhance efforts to detect changes in both seroprevalence and risk behavior.

In summary, these limitations of prevention research may make it difficult for a clinician or program planner to know what interventions would truly be effective. Most studies have been conducted with in-treatment populations, which is a serious limitation to the planner attempting to reach out-of-treatment drug users. Many studies use cross-sectional rather than longitudinal designs, which means that the long-term effects of most interventions are unknown. Finally, almost all studies depend on the self-report of drug users to evaluate outcomes such as needle sharing or unprotected sex. These self-reports may be invalid or unreliable.

SUGGESTIONS FOR DISSEMINATING EFFECTIVE INTERVENTIONS

When a new AIDS prevention technique is developed and proves to be beneficial, its diffusion throughout the AIDS prevention community is by no means automatic. The people who develop the innovations often lack the interest or proficiency to promote the adoption of their improved prevention methods. Practitioners, on the other hand, may not know about better methods, nor will they always be eager to adopt innovations when they first hear about them. In this section, we provide suggestions for the person who has developed a useful AIDS prevention intervention or is interested in seeing that the technique be as widely used as its research results merit.

In the scientist's ideal world, data drive the decision to adopt interventions. Decisions about what approaches to use are made after weighing the evidence on each side. For example, if the goal is to prevent further HIV infection among drug users, the various options for preventing HIV are considered, their effectiveness is estimated, and a decision is made to go with one or more of the interventions. However, real-life decisions do not often work that way, and no matter how convincing research data are, they will not always drive adoption decisions.

Some approaches have appeal, despite evidence that they do not work. For example, public health professionals have known since the anti-venereal-disease campaigns of World War II that fear arousal campaigns are difficult to use effectively (Job, 1988). But the notion still exists that if we could scare people badly enough, they would discontinue the behaviors that are risky for transmitting HIV. In both the United Kingdom and Australia, AIDS education campaigns used "shock tactics" to motivate people to learn more about AIDS. In the United Kingdom, posters and television advertisements emphasized the dangers of AIDS in graphic terms. An evaluation revealed that the fear messages significantly increased anxiety in low-risk students, but not in the drug users who were the target of the campaign (Sherr, 1990). A similar approach in Australia revealed no significant increases in either personal or social concern about AIDS, and levels of knowledge about AIDS did not change (Rigby, Brown, Anagnostou, Ross, & Rosser, 1989). Shock tactics, however, will continue to be attractive to some planners, despite the continuing accumulation of negative evaluation results.

Other decisions are politically complicated. Don Des Jarlais has described the case in which, in 1989, the U.S. Congress nearly banned using federal resources to distribute bleach for needle cleaning or to evaluate such programs (Des Jarlais & Bailey, 1990). An amendment was introduced by both Democrats and Republicans, and it passed because most were not aware of the ways in which these techniques were being used. The bill to which the amendment was attached was then vetoed by the President, but for reasons unrelated to the bleach issue. During reconsideration of the bill, the pro-bleach forces educated congressional staff about the issue and obtained the support of high officials; the final bill that passed did not ban bleach.

Why Disseminate?

Data will never drive policy if policy makers are unaware of the data. However, research-oriented health professionals are seldom involved in bringing their results to the attention of policy makers. A survey of 104 New York City psychologists in academic institutions found that over 70% had at least one research area that could be applied in a real-world setting, but only 20% of the studies were actually applied (Millman, Samet, Shaw, & Braden, 1990). The most frequently identified modalities for communicating information were giving lectures or consulting to organizations; only 11% had communicated with legislators or the judiciary. Data may not be more widely disseminated because universities do not support such activities, because health professionals are not motivated to communicate their findings in other than traditional academic channels, or because they lack the skill to use the available communication channels. In any case, it is uncommon for a research-oriented health professional to bring research findings to the attention of policy makers.

The people who develop and evaluate AIDS prevention techniques should be involved in the dissemination of innovative programs that work. The Institute of Medicine (1989) urges health professionals to educate the public on health issues and to promote the use of scientific information in making decisions. A research-oriented health professional who has evidence that a new intervention is effective should ask the telling question: "If no one knows that I have done it, have I accomplished my goal?" It is the researcher's responsibility to make policy makers aware of research results. Perhaps the researcher's fantasy is that somehow policy makers will come to the scientist. This is unlikely; instead, they respond to the people who approach them. To disseminate interventions that prevent AIDS, effective techniques that encourage policy makers and service providers to talk with each other are needed.

Lessons from the Dissemination Literature

People planning to disseminate effective interventions will exert more influence if they base their dissemination efforts on sound principles. The diffusion of innovations from the research laboratory to the general community has been a topic of interest to some scientists. Glaser, Abelson, and Garrison (1983) have summarized this literature, reviewing more than 2,000 published and unpublished manuscripts on dissemination. The literature on disseminating innovative prevention and treatment techniques, and on encouraging their use, is revealing. Table 10.2 summarizes several key points, which are explained below in more detail.

CLINICIANS READ FEW JOURNAL ARTICLES

Publication in a professional journal is the most traditional way of disseminating the results of an evaluation study, and many efforts at dissemination stop there. However, health professionals do not voraciously read professional journals for guidance in their daily work activities. Clinical psychologists in practice read about two articles per month (Cohen, 1979), and many mental health professionals believe that no research exists that is relevant to their work. Nevertheless, the peer review process of professional publications can screen out exaggerated claims of efficacy, which gives credibility when an evaluation of a program has been published in the professional press. Publication can lead to other dissemination activities, such as listing of the reference in abstract services (e.g., Psychological Abstracts, Social Science Citation Index, or the National Library of Medicine's Medline system). In addition, newsletters can create synopses or abstracts of articles. Finally, the research contributions in some of the most widely read journals, such as the Journal of the American Medical Association (circulation approximately 360,000) and the New England Journal of Medicine (circulation approximately 214,000), are regularly featured in news releases of the mass media.

TABLE 10.2. Suggestions for Disseminating AIDS Prevention Techniques

1. Avoid depending on publications (publications lend credibility to an intervention but may not be widely read)
2. Match technique to target audience
3. Expect programs to modify the intervention
4. Build personal contact with potential adopters

ADOPTION IS NOT RANDOM

What influences whether a program is likely to adopt and use an innovation? In general, the greater the likelihood that an innovation will achieve the desired results, and the more difficult and persistent the problem of concern to a large number of people, the more likely it is to generate interest. DiMaggio and Useem (1979) studied 25 arts organizations in the eastern United States that had adopted innovative organizational policies. Their findings suggest that adoption is most likely to occur (1) when findings confirm the predilections of managers, (2) when an influential person seeks the implementation, and (3) when researchers are involved on a sustained basis in staff deliberations. Innovations are not used when there is a lot of staff turnover in an organization, when the organization does not have the resources to use the findings, and when influential people are hostile or indifferent to the proposed plans. Their study found that the technical quality of a research project had no effect on the likelihood that it would be used!

An intervention will also be more likely to be adopted if it reflects values that are compatible with those of the program considering it. In addition, an intervention that is easy to understand and practical is easier for a program to adopt. In short, AIDS prevention techniques will be more likely to be adopted if they are well matched with the target audience.

ADOPTION IS NOT REPLICATION

Even when a program adopts an intervention it may not do so wholeheartedly or in the way the original developer intended. Rappaport, Seidman, and Davidson (1979) point out that an innovation may be "adopted" by an agency but used in an entirely different way. For example, a program may adopt the ideas of conducting small-group education to prevent AIDS, but may follow a protocol with aims and methods that reflect the background of the agency staff, rather than the innovator's original protocol. The revised intervention may be quite different from the original, so the original study's results are unlikely to be replicated. Despite this drawback, an innovator must expect that a program will modify an intervention, molding it to fit the program's particular situation.

Research Has Compared Dissemination Methods

What techniques can help to spread an effective intervention to the field? Many dissemination techniques have been tried, including printed materials; film, videotapes and audiotapes; consultation; organizational development; on-site technical assistance; network arrangements; and training conferences and workshops.

Although the number of articles about dissemination is large, there have been very few systematic studies of how to encourage the use of techniques in clinical settings. Fairweather and others completed a series of complex experiments in a large-scale effort to disseminate the "community lodge" concept to mental hospitals, using printed materials, workshops, or establishment of a model ward (Fairweather, Sanders, & Tornatzky, 1974; Fairweather, 1980; Tornatzky, Fergus, Avellar, & Fairweather, 1980). The results showed that hospitals were likely to agree to accept the written materials or workshops, but were more likely to adopt the lodge concept if they had agreed to establish a demonstration ward. Later in the study process, those programs that had decided to adopt the lodge concept were randomly assigned to receive either a manual or three visits by consultants. The results showed a significant difference favoring the consultant intervention.

Adoption of innovative methods in substance abuse agencies has been systematically studied in two experiments. In a 2 x 2 factorial design of ways to disseminate program evaluation methods, Stevens and Tornatzky (1980) found superior effectiveness for on-site versus telephone consultations and group versus individual consultations. Another random assignment experiment studied ways of disseminating a job seekers' workshop for patients in 188 drug treatment programs in six U.S. states (Hall, Sorensen, & Loeb, 1988; Sorensen et al., 1988c). It found that 3 months after the dissemination, adoption rates were as follows: site visit at the program, 28%; conference in San Francisco, 19%; printed material (brochure and training manual), 4%; and no-information control, 0%.

In general, these experiments in dissemination indicate that written materials are acceptable to programs, but that adoption is more likely if members of the program staff have received personal contact through a workshop or a technical assistance site visit.

Personal Contact Is Important

A theme of this chapter is that innovators who want others to use their work will need to disseminate it actively through personal contact. The review of Glaser et al. (1983) noted that interactive consultation methods were superior to didactic materials, such as films or printed instructions, as a means of promoting transfer and adoption of new knowledge. This makes sense, in that the process of deploying new technologies is not merely mechanistic; it is a social process that depends on human beings. Health practitioners value and use interpersonal channels more than formal written channels in their practice. They rely on such information sources as nonresearch articles and workshops. In short, the literature on dissemination, including several experimental comparisons of dissemination techniques, indicates that there is no substitute for personal contact.

Personal contact is especially important when cultural groups differ in the behaviors that transmit HIV infection. Chapter 3 of this book pointed out that the cultural context of needle sharing may vary across geographic and ethnic groups. Thus, interventions developed in one community may need to be changed considerably to fit the needs of another community. For example, the cleaning of needles with bleach was first developed as an AIDS prevention technique in San Francisco. In other communities, bleach has not been accepted, but rubbing alcohol has been a workable alternative. Still other groups do not recommend needle cleaning at all, deeming it too closely associated with drug use rather than recovery from addiction.

Suggestions to the Innovator

A successful research project should conclude by disseminating its results. Specially designed diffusion efforts can be conceived, delivered, and evaluated within a systematic research framework. These efforts are likely to be more effective than conventional dissemination techniques, such as publications in professional journals and technical research reports. In short, the innovator should plan the dissemination of research findings, and should evaluate the dissemination techniques.

Dissemination of information among practitioners is achieved by diverse routes. These include the use of media, mail, commission reports, public testimony, workshops, demonstrations of interventions, and site visits to potential adopting programs, as well as the traditional routes of journal publication and presentation at professional conferences.

If an innovator wants research findings to be used by a specific group, it is important to include potential participants or surrogates for them in decision making. This community consultation can help overcome participants' anxiety about adopting a technique, and can help the innovator to revise the technique so that it will be more appropriate to the culture of the participants. Such community consultation has been important in the development of clinical trials research in AIDS (Melton, Levine, Koocher, Rosenthal, & Thompson, 1988), and it will be important in the dissemination of effective ways to prevent AIDS with drug users and their sexual partners.

CONCLUSIONS

This chapter has focused on how to apply scientific knowledge to insure that research-validated AIDS prevention interventions receive widespread support and adoption. For the public health planner, we suggest that selection of an intervention can be based on understanding why drug users and sexual partners engage in AIDS risk behavior. The adopter should weigh the evidence that competing intervention models are effective, depending upon both local reviews of the evidence that projects are effective and the guidelines and suggestions provided by independent review panels. It should be kept in mind that AIDS prevention research is in its infancy; most research has been limited to in-treatment samples, is dependent on self-report, and provides little information about long-term efficacy. In short, many questions remain unanswered. For these reasons, it is essential to build an evaluation component into local AIDS prevention interventions.

State and national organizations should be involved in making judgments about what interventions are worthy, rather than leaving the decisions up to local officials. Professional societies and independent organizations such as the National Academy of Sciences can appoint panels to weigh the evidence that various interventions are effective. These guidelines can help to shape effectiveness of AIDS prevention programs nationwide.

The chapter also has several suggestions for disseminating interventions, based on the lessons of dissemination/utilization research. For the person interested in seeing that an effective intervention gets widespread recognition, we encourage becoming familiar with the findings of this research. In brief, the findings from this area indicate that professional publications are useful but not sufficient for adoption to occur; that innovators should be involved in the dissemination of their work; that planned dissemination efforts can be successful; and that effective dissemination involves person-to-person contact. The Appendix contains more information about resources for learning more about dissemination of effective AIDS prevention interventions.

If dissemination were automatic, this chapter would not be needed. However, there is such an information overload in the AIDS area that it is necessary for the potential adopter of an AIDS prevention technique to select from a dizzying number of competing prevention ideas. For example, the Sixth International Conference on AIDS (San Francisco) had 2,000 presentations; spending 10 minutes at each would take an individual nearly 2 weeks, at 24 hours per day! It is necessary, then, to make judgments about the techniques that best fit a particular situation, and to learn how to promote the interventions that work. Through the twin processes of effective adoption and effective dissemination, the more effective interventions will be more likely to take root, and we will more effectively prevent AIDS among drug abusers and their sexual partners.

Chapter 11

Policy Implications

LAURIE A. WERMUTH
JAMES L. SORENSEN
PATRICIA FRANKS

Rather than marginalizing drug users through the war on drugs, we need to engage them in a war on AIDS.

—AIDS Conference Bulletin, p. 1

The response to AIDS . . . will not be determined strictly by the disease's biological character; rather, that response will be deeply influenced by our social and cultural understanding of disease and its victims. . . . The recognition of the process by which AIDS has been culturally defined provides us with an opportunity to guide and influence responses to the epidemic in ways that will be constructive, effective, and humane.

—Allan M. Brandt (1988, p.163)

This final chapter includes our ideas about what needs to be done to arrest the spread of HIV among drug-injecting individuals and their sexual partners. It begins with a brief profile of the epidemic among injection drug users and their sexual partners; it then provides an overview of needs and remedies for HIV prevention and research among this population.

The AIDS epidemic has brought attention to the largely invisible and stigmatized group of injection drug users in the United States. The practice of drug injection is concentrated among poor and socially marginal groups and is more common among men than women. The exact number of individuals who inject drugs in the United States is unknown, but estimates by various authorities suggest that it is somewhere above 1 million individuals (Institute for Health Policy Studies, 1990, p. 83). Individuals who have injected drugs account for a substantial proportion of AIDS cases to date. Twenty-eight percent of all adult and adolescent AIDS cases reported in the United States from 1981 through late 1989 are attributed to drug injecting among heterosexuals, gay men, and bisexual men. The sexual partners of injection drug users account for an additional 2% of AIDS cases. Judging from the low rates of condom use reported among heterosexual injection drug users, and the long incubation period of HIV, this figure is sure to grow over the next decade.

HIV infection among injection drug users is concentrated in particular geographical areas. Estimates of infection among injection drug users in most cities across the United States range from none to about 20%, whereas in New York City and Newark, New Jersey, the majority of persons who inject drugs are infected. Since underprivileged minority groups are overrepresented among the urban poor, it is not surprising that they are overrepresented among drug injectors and HIV-infected individuals as well. Thus, social class is a factor that shapes the uneven distribution of HIV disease among African-Americans and Latinos in the United States. This concentration is especially striking in cases of AIDS among women and infants. Two-thirds of all U.S. AIDS cases in women and four-fifths of all cases in infants have been among African-Americans and Latinos (Hulley & Hearst, 1989).

The needle sharing that puts injection drug users at risk for transmission of HIV is sometimes the result of necessity and sometimes an expression of solidarity within a subculture. Consequently, rates of infection among needle users are probably also stratified by the social organization of drug use, putting at higher risk those who use "shooting galleries" and engage in collective needle use rituals. It is not clear whether such differences in risky needle practices coincide with higher rates of infection among Latinos and African-Americans. For example, African-American injection drug users in some studies have reported less needle sharing than their white counterparts (Young, Snyder, Friedman, & Myers, 1990; R. E. Fullilove, Golden, Bowser, & Hulley, 1990b). This may reflect the problem of inaccurate self-reports, or it may be a real difference among different social groups' needle use practices. Finally, practices found among whites, Latinos, or African-Americans in one locality may not be found in other places.

The heterosexual spread of HIV in the United States is overwhelmingly concentrated among injection drug users and their sexual partners. Only a minority of injection drug users are regularly using condoms, and in areas with high rates of HIV infection, a new wave of infections most likely is developing. For example, the National Institute on Drug Abuse's National AIDS Demonstration Research (NADR) Project (Rosenshine, 1990) found that among the surveyed 5,280 women who were sexual partners of injection drug users, a majority (62%) reported that their partners never used condoms. There is much that can and should be done to change this situation.

PREVENTION: THE NEED FOR MULTIPLE AND DIVERSE EFFORTS

A variety of simultaneous efforts are needed to slow the spread of HIV among injection drug users and their sexual partners. Table 11.1 lists areas of need and remedies. Injection drug users need education, access to drug treatment, sterile drug use equipment, condoms, and access to HIV antibody testing. Sexual partners of injection drug users, whether they inject drugs themselves or not, need AIDS prevention education, access to substance abuse treatment, and HIV antibody testing. Needs in research include removal of federal restrictions on the study of needle exchange programs; development of shared evaluation standards among AIDS prevention researchers; strategies for improving the reliability of self-report data; study of relapse to risky practices; incorporation of a sociological perspective in study designs and interpretations of data; and attention to interpersonal dynamics in risk behaviors.

Education

Education about preventing the spread of HIV is most effective if information is available from a variety of sources and venues. Print and broadcast media, brochures, billboards, and videos provide information that can alert individuals to risk and dispel misconceptions. Through newspaper and radio coverage of pediatric AIDS cases and the spread of HIV through drug injection and sexual relationships, media have alerted many to the dangers they face. Widely broadcast messages that contain explicit information about HIV and its transmission can alert and inform the public.

Media Campaigns

Injection drug users and their female sexual partners have been targeted in small-scale media efforts such as video presentations and brochures presented in medical clinics. More widespread media campaigns have been aimed at gay men and heterosexuals in general. These messages, however, do not adequately address the fact that monogamy is not a solution for women whose partners inject drugs.

HIV education programs in substance abuse treatment programs can reinforce the positive efforts of drug and alcohol abusers to prevent the spread of HIV. Clients also develop social support among their peers and counselors for changing sex and drug use practices.

Media campaigns can raise public consciousness about protection against HIV, and in particular about condom use. There perhaps has

TABLE 11.1. HIV Prevention with Injection Drug Abusers and Their Sexual Partners

Areas of need	Remedies
Education	Targeted media campaigns Other programs
Drug treatment	Expansion of programs and services Care of HIV-infected clients
Access to: Sterile injection equipment Condoms HIV antibody testing	Through: Outreach programs Community-based health clinics Drug treatment programs
Research	Removal of restrictions against studying syringe exchanges Development of evaluation standards Improvement of self-report data Study of relapse A sociological perspective Attention to interpersonal dynamics

been an overemphasis, however, on targeting women, instructing them to persuade their partners to use condoms. This inadvertently sexist approach also appears in directives encouraging researchers to find "ways that women can get their men to wear condoms" (Cohen, Hauer, & Wofsy, 1989).

A positively focused and aggressive campaign to promote condom use among heterosexual men is needed. Men can be encouraged to use condoms for both altruistic and self-protective purposes. This can be done in a variety of ways: through outreach workers, in the schools, by health and drug treatment clinicians, and in the media. A variety of male role models (from sports heroes to respected community leaders) can speak to men, suggesting that condom use is worth the protection afforded to oneself and loved ones. Depending on the medium, such messages can include explicit information about how to use condoms correctly, as well as the suggestion to experiment with a variety of kinds until a preferred one is found.

Fear by itself is not necessarily helpful in bringing about changed sexual or drug use practices. Frightening information and pictures without instructions on how to take positive action may succeed only in creating anxiety. Without becoming overly sentimental, clinical, or moralistic, prevention messages can offer explicit directions regarding how to prevent HIV transmission. Messages can tap both altruistic and self-protective motives, and can speak openly of the value of saving human lives.

Outreach Programs

The term "outreach" has come to describe the efforts to reach individuals in their own environment with HIV prevention information and supplies. Outreach programs have concentrated their efforts in "high-risk" neighborhoods. Grassroots efforts or specially funded projects that employ "insiders" are able to reach groups that may not otherwise be aware of the problem and their personal risk, or may not have access to preventive supplies. Operating on the turf of those at risk, outreach workers can gain the trust of individuals and provide condoms, bleach bottles, or sterile drug-injecting equipment. Outreach workers can also give counsel and encouragement to "stay safe." A more difficult task for outreach workers is to persuade heterosexual men to use condoms—not just with prostitutes and casual sexual partners, but with their wives and steady sexual partners as well.

Despite the positive advances that have been made by outreach efforts, there is still much to be done. Just at the time that funding is decreasing, more and diversified outreach projects are needed. The National Institute on Drug Abuse has discontinued its multisite demonstration outreach project to injection drug abusers and sexual partners, and there is little funding available to institutionalize these programs within existing agencies and organizations. Indeed, many smaller programs are having to curtail their services in the face of contracting budgets and increased demands resulting from the epidemic.

Poor inner-city minority communities will suffer most dearly from the lack of funds for outreach programs. Consequently, local voluntary efforts through grassroots organizations, businesses, and churches may hold the greatest hope for keeping the spread of HIV infection in check. Minority communities in which the virus has spread more rapidly than other areas require indigenous outreach workers to work through local organizations, as well as on the streets. Outreach workers can attempt work "from the ground up" to lobby for the needs of those they serve by attending community and agency meetings, speaking to the media, and otherwise lobbying for their constituencies. Such efforts can have the positive effect of reducing stigma, creating access to services, and establishing links to those with decision-making power. It is also possible for groups of prostitutes and drug injectors to be organized into self-help groups, empowering changes and generating decision-making power of their own (Friedman et al., 1990). Grassroots community organizing has the potential to raise awareness, exercise political clout, and provide the support needed to sustain individual and group efforts to avoid HIV risk (Shaw, 1988). But however powerful the potential of grassroots efforts, they cannot be sustained without funding and institutional support.

If another wave of federal funding for AIDS prevention and research were initiated, outreach activities could slow the spread of HIV. Among young gay men, drug injectors, and the sexual partners of both these groups, indigenously staffed outreach efforts could have a significant impact.

Drug Treatment

Addicted individuals have difficulty taking precautions against HIV infection. The frequent use of drugs and alcohol in sexual liaisons impedes the consistent use of condoms and sterile needles. Drug and alcohol use as a prelude to sex has been found to be associated with unprotected intercourse and has been dubbed "chemical foreplay" by one group of researchers (R. E. Fullilove et al., 1990b).

Drug treatment clinics play a central role in educating and promoting changes in drug use and sexual norms, and in counseling clients about their risk. More clinics and more treatment slots within existing clinics are needed, and ready entry to detoxification programs is essential in preventing the transmission of HIV.

While they are in treatment programs, individuals find it easier to reduce or refrain from needle use. Treatment programs are also avenues for distributing information and providing voluntary HIV antibody testing. Receiving counseling and HIV antibody testing assists drug users in the process of coming to grips with AIDS risk, and often in gaining awareness of possible transmission to their sexual partners. Clinical settings provide a forum for drug users to collectively devise strategies for avoiding risks, and to evolve safer norms for needle use and sexual practices.

Treatment programs are available in many urban areas, but they offer only a partial solution to HIV prevention. Existing programs do not have enough treatment openings to meet demand, and not all drug injectors desire methadone treatment. In addition, while methadone provides a legal substitute for heroin, there is no such pharmacological remedy for cocaine or amphetamine use. For persons who have stopped drug use, the Twelve-Step self-help programs of Narcotics Anonymous, Cocaine Anonymous, and Alcoholics Anonymous are supportive and HIV-preventive remedies.

As discussed in Chapter 6, the care of HIV-infected individuals in drug treatment requires flexibility, intensive counseling, and comprehensive case management. It is important that HIV-infected individuals not be segregated from other clients, yet receive the daily attention they need. Provision of drug treatment in itself enhances individuals' chances of maintaining their health; it also makes possible the treatment of medical problems and delivery of assistance with practical difficulties. Patients can benefit from coordination (and proximity when possible) of care by drug treatment and HIV medical staff. Maintaining a more flexible treatment protocol for HIV-symptomatic patients to help prevent relapse is a sound policy for both patients and the public health. Unfortunately, limited funds for drug treatment and growing numbers of ill clients in methadone clinics are putting pressure on clinics and constraining their abilities to meet the needs of HIV-infected clients.

When possible, drug treatment programs can assist HIV-infected patients with the multiple problems they face. Clients may need help with housing, welfare arrangements, meals, transportation, and health care. They need education about HIV and daily medical observation. HIV-infected clients can also benefit from self-help groups, supportive psychotherapy, and (when needed) the use of psychiatric medications.

Treatments for cocaine abuse are sorely needed both within methadone programs and in independent programs. In addition, women in treatment programs need gynecological care and birth control counseling. All clients need information about preventing the spread of sexually transmitted diseases, including training in the proper use of condoms. Liaison to other services is also helpful for needs such as job training, parenting education, and self-help programs. In these ways, programs can assist drug injectors in "mainstreaming" their lives and thus can help to prevent relapse (Marlatt & Gordon, 1985).

Treatment clinic waiting lists are not a humane response to HIV-infected individuals or drug-dependent individuals in general. If treatment is not available when an addicted person arrives at the door, an opportunity is lost to prevent the spread of HIV. Those clients in detoxification programs who wish to remain in treatment should be able to do so. Additional treatment spaces, counseling, and medical staff are needed to meet these needs. Such an expansion of programming would be sound HIV prevention policy. It would save lives and money by preventing many drug abusers from becoming infected and ill with HIV disease.

Drug treatment programs also provide an opportunity to reach and counsel the sexual partners of injection drug users about their HIV risk. HIV-infected clients can be given the option of informing their partners, or they may choose to have the local health department notify their sexual partners. Partner notification programs are essential to help slow the spread of the virus and to provide individuals exposed to the virus with access to information, testing, and (if needed) medical care. It is our opinion, however, that partner notification should never be a prerequisite to gaining access to drug treatment, medical care, or participation in research projects. Such policies have the counterproductive effect of dissuading individuals from receiving the care they need, and thereby they directly impede HIV prevention.

Access to Sterile Injection Equipment, Condoms, and HIV Antibody Testing

Outreach programs are effective in dispensing information, small bleach bottles, and condoms to drug users and their sexual partners. Needle exchange programs also make it possible for individuals to exchange their used equipment for new, sterile needles and syringes. These programs are run by local activists and are often illegal. If these efforts were made legal, it is possible that they could further slow the spread of HIV among drug users and their sexual partners. In addition, pharmacies could dispense sterile needles to drug users as they now do to hemophiliacs. Community health clinics, drug treatment programs, and HIV antibody testing programs can also make available instructions for safe sex and drug use, as well as condoms and bleach bottles.

Public health agencies and condom manufacturers can assist in HIV prevention by providing subsidized or discounted supplies of condoms. These could be distributed at drug treatment clinics, at clinics treating sexually transmitted diseases, and by outreach programs. Inexpensive supplies of condoms also could be sold to local departments of public health for free distribution in "high-risk" neighborhoods. Cooperation among community leaders, grassroots activists, and public health personnel can facilitate making supplies for safer sex and drug use accessible.

Programs for HIV antibody testing have a central role to play in preventing the spread of infection. Many individuals are unaware of their HIV-infected status and their ability to transmit the virus to others. Testing programs that include pre- and posttest counseling help individuals to learn more about HIV disease, how it is transmitted, and whether they are infected. Substance abuse treatment programs and community clinics often provide HIV antibody testing. Many individuals acknowledge and discuss their risk for the first time when being tested. With the help of trained counselors, individuals can get support and the information necessary to refrain from risky sexual and drug use practices. The availability of anonymous testing is important in attracting those individuals who do not wish to have their identity revealed.

Research

1. Federal restrictions on the evaluation of syringe exchanges should be lifted, so that well-designed trials can be conducted. It has long been necessary to study certain illegal activities in order for the public health to be served. Anal sex and prostitution are illegal in many parts of the United States, and yet it has been essential that we investigate the sexual practices associated with the spread of HIV disease. The same is the case for programs that provide the exchange of syringes. If need be, funding for evaluation studies could begin with legal needle exchange programs, such as those in Tacoma and Seattle. Moreover, syringe exchanges present some special methodological advantages for evaluation, in that most can supplement self-reported data with data on the returned syringes. For example, syringes have been analyzed for the presence of HIV antibodies in studies in Australia (Wolk et al., 1988). Furthermore, syringe exchanges offer the potential to reach groups of injection drug users who have not thus far been reached in treatment programs. We believe it is shortsighted to refuse to evaluate exchange programs, for there is no other way to discover their true effects.

2. Standards must be developed to evaluate the efficacy of AIDS prevention research. These standards can take into account the balance of methodological difficulties and importance of the preventive intervention being evaluated. The standards can be used to gauge the quality of planned and existing research. They will aid the application of scientific principles, rather than solely relying on what the community will readily support or on political expedience in determining the interventions that slow the spread of AIDS. The National Research Council has made an excellent start at developing these standards with the publication of Evaluating AIDS Prevention Programs (Coyle, Boruch, & Turner, 1989, 1990), which makes recommendations for the evaluation of community-based interventions and HIV testing programs.

3. Ways must be found to improve the quality of self-reported data regarding drug use and AIDS risk behaviors. A recent report of the National Academy of Sciences suggests that such research must consider the problems introduced by nonresponse factors, along with such issues as the effects of anonymity guarantees on survey responses, the effects of question wording and context, and the effects of asking respondents to recall different time periods (Miller, Turner, & Moses, 1990, p. 33).

4. Research should focus on the motivations that drive people to continue with risky behaviors. Friedman and Des Jarlais (1989) point out that it is important to design studies that distinguish between the drug users' intent to protect themselves from infection and their intent to protect others from outward transmission. For example, a drug user

may clean a needle before using it to protect himself or herself, then pass it on to a "shooting partner" without cleaning it. Although needle use behavior differs somewhat in this respect from sexual behavior, there too we need to begin to distinguish between altruistic and self-protective safer sex practices. Both kinds of motivation need to be stressed and encouraged in intervention studies.

5. Research should also focus on the reasons why people relapse to risky behaviors some time after they have adopted safe practices. In one study, over a third of the injection drug users who reported that they had changed their behaviors because of AIDS also reported that they had not maintained AIDS risk reduction (Des Jarlais, Tross, Abdul-Quader, Kouzi, & Friedman, 1989b). Similarly, Stall, Ekstrand, Pollack, and Coates (1990a) found that 19% of their sample of gay men in a follow-up survey reported relapse to high-risk sex after they had reported having only safe sex at a previous interview. Methods are already well developed to help to prevent relapse to drug and alcohol abuse; for an example, see Marlatt and Gordon (1985). A key direction for research is to develop interventions that prevent relapse to high-risk behaviors for transmitting HIV.

6. A sociological perspective is needed in AIDS behavioral research. Factors of socioeconomic class, interpersonal relationships, gender dynamics, and ethnic/racial cultures have thus far been neglected. Too often, the analysis of AIDS risk and the measurement of behavioral outcomes (e.g., in intervention studies) are reduced to discrete and individual "risk behaviors." This approach often blinds investigators to the cultural and social-structural factors that place particular social groups at greater risk for HIV. In addition, measurement of risk in heterosexual relationships often does not reflect the asymmetry of control over condom use for men and women. Moreover, because acquiring an HIV infection occurs now nearly exclusively in specific behavioral contexts, there is an urgent need to conceptualize risk in those interpersonal and social contexts. Our studies should examine relationships as a key variable, paying attention to their duration, behavioral norms, level of commitment, emotional and material connectedness, and level of dependency.

7. More studies should address the interpersonal context of safer sex among heterosexuals. Few studies have dealt with these issues. An exception is a study by Magura, Shapiro, Siddiqi, and Lipton (1990), which found that condom use among intravenous drug users was independently associated with greater personal acceptance of condoms, greater partner receptivity to sexual protection, and recent entry to methadone treatment. In addition, Worth (1989) has pointed out that the ability of women to introduce condom use to their male partners is

dependent on relative sexual equality between men and women. Moreover, changes in couples' sex lives require sensitive negotiations. The proposal to adopt condom use affects more than the mechanics of having sex; it may provoke accusations or violence and threats to end relationships. Difficulties arise from the fact that condoms are a male-controlled method over which women can exercise influence but not direct control. When women are faced with partners who refuse to use condoms, economic and emotional dependence may make it difficult for these women (especially those with children) to leave relationships (Mays & Cochran, 1988). Women need female-controlled methods of HIV prevention (Stein, 1990). These issues call for attention in AIDS prevention and research activities.

CONCLUSIONS

As we have seen among gay men in San Francisco, well-planned and culturally appropriate campaigns can affect dramatic changes in HIV risk behavior (Winkelstein et al., 1988). San Francisco's communities of gay men have demonstrated that grassroots organizing, mutual support for healthy practices, and group solidarity can slow the spread of HIV and influence the development of policies at the local, state, and national levels. Although drug injectors and their sexual partners differ dramatically from this group, there are useful lessons to be learned for activists and researchers: Solutions must come from within local cultures, and resources must be given to agencies and individuals best equipped to influence change. Responding positively with methods that support the adoption of safe practices will have more lasting and effective value than will punitive measures. In addition, collaboration among local activists, public health personnel, and researchers is necessary both for sound programs and for research. This approach holds greatest promise in reshaping the ideological context of AIDS prevention among individuals who inject drugs and among their sexual partners. With sustained effort, these individuals may move away from being characterized by "vectors of disease" and toward becoming a mobilized group with a legitimate voice for their needs in the battle against HIV disease.

References

Abdul-Quader, A., Tross, S., Des Jarlais, D. C., Kouzi, A., Friedman, S. R., & McCoy, E. (1989, June). *Predictors of attempted sexual behavior change in a street sample of active male IV drug users in New York City*. Poster presented at the Fifth International Conference on AIDS, Montreal.

Adair Films. (1985). *AIDS antibody testing at alternative sites* [videotape]. San Francisco: San Francisco AIDS Foundation/San Francisco Department of Public Health.

AIDS Conference Bulletin. (1990, June). *Stimson: Enlist drug users to fight AIDS*. Sixth International Conference on AIDS, San Francisco.

Alberto, S. (1990, June). *Incidence of seroconversion (SC) in women who are steady partners of HIV infected men (IC)*. Poster presented at the Sixth International Conference on AIDS, San Francisco.

Amaro, H. (1988). Considerations for prevention of HIV infection among Hispanic women. *Psychology of Women Quarterly, 12*, 429443.

Amsel, Z., Battjes, R., & Pickens, R. (1990, June). *Cocaine use and HIV risk among intravenous opiate addicts*. Poster presented at the Sixth International Conference on AIDS, San Francisco.

Amsel, Z., Mandell, W., Matthias, L., Mason, C., & Hocherman, I. (1976). Reliability and validity self-reported illegal activities and drug use collected from narcotic addicts. *International Journal of the Addictions, 11*, 325–336.

Arndt, I., Dorozynsky, L., Woody, G., McLellan, A., & O'Brien, C. (1988). Desipramine treatment of cocaine abuse in methadone maintained outpatients. In L. S. Harris (Ed.), *Problems of drug dependence, 1988 (NIDA Research Monograph Series No. 90*, DHHS Publication No. ADM 89-1605, p. 347). Washington, DC: U.S. Government Printing Office. (Abstract)

Arnold, C. B. (1972). The sexual behavior of inner city adolescent condom users. *Journal of Sex Research, 8*, 298309.

Baldwin, J. D., & Baldwin, J. I. (1988). Factors affecting AIDS related sexual risk-taking behavior among college students. *Journal of Sex Research, 25*, 181–196.

Ball, J. C., Lange, W., Myers, C., & Friedman, S. (1988). Reducing the risk of AIDS through methadone maintenance treatment. *Journal of Health and Social Behavior, 29*, 214–226.

Bandura, A. (1977). Self-efficacy: Toward a unifying theory of behavior change. *Psychological Review, 84*, 191–215.

Bandura, A. (1989). Perceived self-efficacy in the exercise of control over AIDS infection. In V. M. Mays, G. W. Albee, & S. F. Schneider (Eds.), *Primary prevention of AIDS: Psychological approaches* (pp. 128–141). Newbury Park, CA: Sage.

Bandura, A. (1990). Perceived self-efficacy in the exercise of control over AIDS infection. *Evaluation and Program Planning, 13*, 9–17.

Batki, S. L. (1988). Treatment of intravenous drug users with AIDS: The role of methadone maintenance. *Journal of Psychoactive Drugs, 20*, 213–216.

Batki, S. L. (1990). Buspirone in drug users with AIDS or AIDS-related condition. *Journal of Clinical Psychopharmacology, 10*(Suppl), 111S–115S.

Batki, S. L., London, J., Goosby, E., Clement, M., Wolfe, R., Ryan, C., French, D., Young, M., Miller, D., Christmas, R., & Sorensen, J. (1990a, June). *Medical care for intravenous drug users with AIDS and ARC: Delivering services at a methadone treatment program.* Paper presented at the Sixth International Conference on AIDS, San Francisco.

Batki, S. L., Manfredi, L., & Dumontet, R. (1990b). Problems with group therapy for cocaine abuse in HIV-infected methadone patients. *Alcoholism: Clinical and Experimental Research, 14*, 135. (Abstract)

Batki, S. L., Manfredi, L., Sorensen, J., Jacob, P., Dumontet, R., & Jones, R. T. (1991). Fluoxetine for cocaine abuse in methadone patients: Preliminary findings. In L. S. Harris (Ed.), *Problems of drug dependence, 1990 (NIDA Research Monograph Series* No. 15, DHHS Publication No. ADM 91-1753, pp. 516–517). Washington, DC: U.S. Government Printing Office. (Abstract)

Batki, S. L., Sorensen, J., Coates, C., & Gibson, D. (1988a). Methadone maintenance for AIDS-affected IV drug users: Treatment outcome and psychiatric factors after three months. In L. S. Harris (Ed.), *Problems of drug dependence, 1988 (NIDA Research Monograph Series No. 90*, DHHS Publication No. ADM 89-1605, p. 343). Washington, DC: U.S. Government Printing Office. (Abstract)

Batki, S. L., Sorensen, J., Faltz, B., & Madover, S. (1988b). AIDS among intravenous drug users: Psychiatric aspects of treatment. *Hospital and Community Psychiatry, 39*, 439–441.

Batki, S. L., Sorensen, J., Gibson, D., & Maude-Griffin, P. (1990c). HIV-infected IV drug users in methadone treatment: Outcome and psychological correlates—a preliminary report. In L. S. Harris (Ed.), *Problems of drug dependence, 1989 (NIDA Research Monograph Series No. 95*, DHHS Publication No. ADM 90-1663, pp. 405406). Washington, DC: U.S. Government Printing Office. (Abstract)

Battjes, R. J., & Pickens, R. (1988, June). *AIDS transmission behavior among intravenous drug users.* Poster presented at the Fourth International Conference on AIDS, Stockholm.

Bean, C. (1989). The minority AIDS project: Dealing with AIDS in a black community in Los Angeles. In *AIDS and intravenous drug abuse among minorities* (DHHS Publication No. ADM 90-1637, pp. 45–49). Washington, DC: U.S. Government Printing Office.

Beck, A. T., & Frankel, A. (1981). A conceptualization of threat communications and protective health behavior. *Social Psychology Quarterly, 44*, 204–217.

Beck, A. T., Ward, C. H., Mendelson, M., Mock, J., & Erbaugh, J. (1961). An inventory for measuring depression. *Archives of General Psychiatry, 4,* 561–571.

Beck, A. T., Weissman, A., Lester, D., & Trexler, L. (1975). The measurement of pessimism: The Hopelessness Scale. *Journal of Consulting and Clinical Psychology, 42,* 861–865.

Becker, M. H. (1974). The health belief model and personal health behavior. *Health Education Monographs, 2,* 220–243.

Becker, M. H., & Joseph, J. G. (1988). AIDS and behavior change to reduce risk: A review. *American Journal of Public Health, 78,* 394–410.

Belle, D. (1990). Poverty and women's mental health. *American Psychologist, 45,* 385–389.

Ben-Yehuda, N. (1990). *The politics and morality of deviance: Moral panics, drug abuse, deviant science, and reversed stigmatization.* Albany: State University of New York.

Bixler, R. E., Palacios-Jiminez, L., & Springer, E. (1987). *AIDS prevention for substance abuse treatment programs.* (Available from Narcotics and Drug Research, Inc., 251 New Karner Road, Albany, NY 12205)

Blizinsky, M., & Reid, W. (1980). Problem focus and change in a brief treatment model. *Social Work, 25,* 89–92.

Bodenheimer, H., Fulton, J., & Kramer, P. (1986). Acceptance of hepatitis B vaccine among hospital workers. *American Journal of Public Health, 76,* 252–255.

Bolland, K., & Hunter, A. (1990). *Seattle needle exchange resource manual.* (Available from the Needle Exchange and IDU Advocate Committee, ACT-UP/Seattle, 1206 Pike St., Suite 814, Seattle, WA 98122)

Brandt, A. B. (1988). AIDS: From social history to social policy. In E. F. Fee & D. M. Fox (Eds.), *AIDS: The burdens of history* (pp. 147–171). Berkeley: University of California Press.

Breitman, P., Knutson, K., & Reed, P. (1987). *How to get your lover to use a condom and why you should.* New York: Prima Publishing/St. Martins Press.

Brown, L. S., Chu, A., Nemoto, T., Ajuluchukwu, D., & Primm, B. (1989). Human immunodeficiency virus infection in a cohort of intravenous drug users in NYC: Demographic, behavioral, and clinical features. *New York State Journal of Medicine, 320,* 1493–1494.

Brown, L. S., Murphy, D. L., & Primm, B. J. (1987). Needle sharing and AIDS in U. S. minorities [letter]. *Journal of the American Medical Association, 258,* 1474–1475.

Brown, L. S., & Primm, B. J. (1989). A perspective on the spread of AIDS among minority intravenous drug abusers. In *AIDS and intravenous drug abuse among minorities* (DHHS Publication No. ADM 90-1637, pp. 323). Washington, DC: U.S. Government Printing Office.

Brownell, K. D., Marlatt, G. A., Lichtenstein, E., & Wilson, G. T. (1986). Understanding and preventing relapse. *American Psychologist, 7,* 765– 782.

Buffum, J. (1988). Substance abuse and high risk sexual behavior: Drugs and sex—the dark side. *Journal of Psychoactive Drugs, 20,* 165–168.

Calsyn, D. A., & Saxon, A. J. (1987). A system for uniform application of contingencies for illicit drug use. *Journal of Substance Abuse Treatment, 4,* 41–47.

Calsyn, D. A., Saxon, A. J., & Freeman, G. (1990, June). *Correlates of HIV risk reduction among IVDUs*. Poster presented at the Sixth International Conference on AIDS, San Francisco.

Casadonte, P. P., Des Jarlais, D. C., Friedman, S. R., & Rotrosen, J. (1988, June). *Psychological and behavioral impact of learning HIV test results in IV drug users*. Poster presented at the Fourth International AIDS Conference, Stockholm.

Casadonte, P. P., Des Jarlais, D. C., Smith, T., Novatt, A., & Herndal, P. (1986, June). *Psychological and behavioral impact of learning HTLV-III/LAV antibody test results*. Paper presented at the Second International Conference on AIDS, Paris.

Catania, J. A., Kegeles, S., & Coates, T. J. (1990). Toward an understanding of risk behavior: An AIDS risk-reduction model. *Health Education Quarterly, 17*, 53–92.

Catania, J., Kegeles, S., & Coates, T. (1988, June). *Seeking help for problems in reducing high-risk sexual behavior*. Paper presented at the Fourth International Conference on AIDS, Stockholm.

Catania, J. A., McDermott, L. J., & Wood, J. A. (1984). Assessment of locus of control: Situational specificity in the sexual context. *Journal of Sex Research, 20*, 310–324.

Centers for Disease Control (CDC). (1984, January). *HIV/AIDS surveillance report*, Atlanta: Author.

Centers for Disease Control (CDC). (1987). Human immunodeficiency virus in the United States. *Morbidity and Mortality Weekly Report, 36*, 801–804.

Centers for Disease Control (CDC). (1989). AIDS and human immunodeficiency virus infection in the United States: 1988 update. *Morbidity and Mortality Weekly Report*, 38(S-4), 1–38.

Centers for Disease Control (CDC). (1990a, January). *HIV/AIDS surveillance report*. Atlanta: Author.

Centers for Disease Control (CDC). (1990b, December). *HIV/AIDS surveillance report*. Atlanta: Author.

Centers for Disease Control (CDC). (1991, January). *HIV/AIDS surveillance report*. Atlanta: Author.

Chaisson, R. E., Bacchetti, P., Osmond, D., Brodie, B., Sande, M. A., & Moss, A. R. (1989). Cocaine use and HIV infection in intravenous drug users in San Francisco. *Journal of the American Medical Association, 261*, 561–565.

Chaisson, R. E., Moss, A. R., Onishi, R., Osmond, D., & Carlson, J. R. (1987a). Human immunodeficiency virus infection in heterosexual intravenous drug users in San Francisco. *American Journal of Public Health, 77*, 169–171.

Chaisson, R. E., Osmond, D., Moss, A. R., Feldman, H. W., & Biernacki, P. (1987b). HIV, bleach, and needle sharing [letter]. *Lancet, i*, 1430.

Chambers, C. D., Taylor, W. J. R., & Moffett, A. D. (1972). The incidence of cocaine use among methadone maintenance patients. *International Journal of the Addictions, 7*, 427–441.

Chitwood, D. D., McCoy, C. B., Inciardi, J. A., McBride, D. C., Comerford, M., Trapido, E., McCoy, V., Page, J. B., Griffin, J., Fletcher, M. A., & Ashman, M. A. (1990a). HIV seropositivity of needles from shooting galleries in South Florida. *American Journal of Public Health, 80*, 150–152.

Chitwood, D. D., McCoy, C. B., McCoy, H. V., McKay, C., McBride, D. C., & Comerford, M. (1990b, June). *Evaluation of a risk reduction program for intravenous drug users.* Poster presented at the Sixth International Conference on AIDS, San Francisco.

Choi, K.-H., Wermuth, L., & Sorensen, J. (1990, June). *Predictors of condoms use among women sexual partners of intravenous drug users.* Poster presented at the Sixth International Conference on AIDS, San Francisco.

Clark, G. L., Downing, M., McQuie, H., Gann, D., Dietrich, R., Case, P., Haber, J., & Fergusson, B. (1989, June). *Street based needle exchange programs: The next step in HIV prevention.* Poster presented at the Fifth International Conference on AIDS, Montreal.

Cleary, P., Rogers. T., Singer, E., Avorn, J., Devanter, N., Perry, S., & Pindyck, J. (1986). Health education about AIDS among seropositive blood donors. *Health Education Quarterly, 13*, 317–329.

Coates, T. J., Stall, R., Kegeles, S. M., Lo, B., Marin, S. F., & McKusick, L. (1988). AIDS antibody testing: Will it stop the AIDS epidemic, will it help people infected with HIV? *American Psychologist, 43*, 859–864.

Cochran, S. D. (1989). *Women and HIV infection: Issues in prevention and behavior change.* In V. M. Mays, G. W. Albee, & S. F. Schneider (Eds.), Primary prevention of AIDS: Psychological approaches (pp. 309–327). Newbury Park, CA: Sage.

Cohen, L. H. (1979). The research readership and information source reliance of clinical psychologists. *Professional Psychology, 10*, 780–785.

Cohen, J. B., Alexander, P., & Wofsy, C. B. (1988). Prostitutes and AIDS: Public policy issues. *AIDS and Public Policy Journal, 3*, 16–22.

Cohen, J. B., Hauer, L. B., & Wofsy, C. B. (1989). Women and IV drugs: Parenteral and heterosexual transmission of human immunodeficiency virus. *Journal of Drug Issues, 19*, 39–56.

Coleman, B. (1990, July 11). AIDS moving up list as cause of death for women. *San Francisco Examiner*, p. A9.

Collins, R. (1975). *Conflict sociology.* New York: Academic Press.

Council on Scientific Affairs, American Medical Association. (1989). Reducing transmission of human immunodeficiency virus (HIV) among and through intravenous drug users. *AIDS and Public Policy Journal, 4*, 142–151.

Cox, C. P., Selwyn, P. A., Schoenbaum, E. E., O'Dowd, M. A., & Drucker, E. (1986). *Psychological and behavioral consequences of HTLV-III/LAV antibody testing and notification among intravenous drug users in a methadone program in New York.* Paper presented at the Second International Conference on AIDS, Paris.

Coyle, S. L., Boruch, R. F., & Turner, C. F. (Eds.). (1989). *Evaluating AIDS prevention programs.* Washington, DC: National Academy Press.

Coyle, S. L., Boruch, R. F., & Turner, C. F. (Eds.). (1990). *Evaluating AIDS prevention programs (expanded ed.).* Washington, DC: National Academy Press.

Crespo, H. (1989). AIDS prevention directed at Hispanic youths and families in large American cities. In *AIDS and intravenous drug abuse among minori-*

ties (DHHS Publication No. ADM 90-1637, pp. 50–54). Washington, DC: U.S. Government Printing Office.

Curtis, J. L., Crummery, F. C., Baker, S. N., Foster, R. E., Khanyile, C. S., & Wilkins, R. (1989). HIV screening and counseling for intravenous drug abuse patients: Staff and patient attitudes. *Journal of the American Medical Association, 261*, 258–262.

Dackis, C. A., Gold, M., Davies, R., & Sweeney, D. R. (1985–1986). Bromocriptine treatment for cocaine abuse: The dopamine depletion hypothesis. *International Journal of Psychiatry in Medicine, 15*, 125–135.

Darrow, W. W. (1974). Attitudes toward condom use and the acceptance of venereal disease prophylactics. In M. H. Redford, G. W. Duncan, & D. J. Prager (Eds.), *The condom: Increasing utilization in the United States* (pp. 173–185). San Francisco: San Francisco Press.

De Leon, G. (1984). *The therapeutic community: Study of effectiveness* (DHHS Publication No. ADM 84-1286). Washington, DC: U.S. Government Printing Office.

Derby, S. B., & Lovelle-Drache, J. M. (1990, December). *Perception of risk-taking among women at high risk for HIV*. Paper presented at the UCSF Tenth Annual Internal Medicine Research Conference, San Francisco.

Des Jarlais, D. C. (1988a). *The effectiveness of AIDS educational programs for intravenous drug users*. Paper prepared for the U.S. Office of Technology Assessment.

Des Jarlais, D. C. (1988b, June). *HIV infection among persons who inject illicit drugs: Problems and progress*. Paper presented at the Fourth International Conference on AIDS, Stockholm.

Des Jarlais, D. C. (1990). Stages in the response of the drug abuse treatment system to the AIDS epidemic in New York City. *Journal of Drug Issues, 20*, 335–347.

Des Jarlais, D. C., & Bailey, W. (1990, June). *Almost banning bleach: An empirical study of AIDS policy development in the U.S.* Paper presented at the Sixth International Conference on AIDS, San Francisco.

Des Jarlais, D. C., Chamberland, M. E., Yancovitz, S. R., Weinberg, P., & Friedman, S. R. (1984). Heterosexual partners: A large risk group for AIDS. *Lancet*, 1346–1347.

Des Jarlais, D. C., & Friedman, S. R. (1988). The psychology of preventing AIDS among intravenous drug users: A social learning conceptualization. *American Psychologist, 43*, 865–870.

Des Jarlais, D. C., Friedman, S. R., Casriel, C., & Kott, A. (1987a). AIDS and preventing initiation into intravenous (IV) drug use. *Psychology and Health, 1*, 179–194.

Des Jarlais, D. C., Friedman, S. R., & Hopkins, W. (1985). Risk reduction for the acquired immunodeficiency syndrome among drug users. *Annals of Internal Medicine, 103*, 755–759.

Des Jarlais, D. C., Friedman, S. R., Marmor, M., Cohen, H., Mildvan, D., Yancovitz, S., Mathur, U., El-Sadr, W., Spira, T., Garber, J., Beatrice, S., Abdul-Quader, A., & Sotheran, J. (1987b). Development of AIDS, HIV seroconversion, and potential cofactors for T4 cell loss in a cohort of intravenous drug users. *AIDS, 1*, 105–111.

Des Jarlais, D. C., Friedman, S. R., Novick, D. M., Sotheran, J. L., Thomas, P., Yancovitz, S. R., Mildvan, D., Weber, J., Kreek, M. J., Maslansky, R., Bartelme, S., Spira, T., & Marmor, M. (1989a). HIV-1 infection among intravenous drug users in Manhattan, New York City, from 1977 through 1987. *Journal of the American Medical Association, 261*, 1008–1012.

Des Jarlais, D. C., & Hopkins, W. (1985). Free needles for intravenous drug users at risk for AIDS: Current developments in New York City [Letter]. *New England Journal of Medicine, 313*, 1476.

Des Jarlais, D. C., Tross, S., Abdul-Quader, A., Kouzzi, A., & Friedman, S. R. (1989b, June). *Intravenous drug users and the maintenance of behavior change.* Paper presented at the Fifth International Conference on AIDS, Montreal.

Dilley, J., Seymour, N., & Eya, E. (1987). *Guidelines for disclosing AIDS antibody test results.* San Francisco: University of California AIDS Health Project.

DiMaggio, P., & Useem, M. (1979). Decentralized applied research: Factors affecting the use of audience research by arts organizations. *Journal of Applied Behavioral Science, 15*, 79–94.

Donoghoe, M., Dolan, K., & Stimson, G. (1990, June). *An evaluation of the further development of syringe-exchanges in England.* Poster presented at the Sixth International Conference on AIDS, San Francisco.

Drucker, E. (1986). AIDS and addiction in New York City. *American Journal of Alcohol and Drug Abuse, 12*, 165–181.

D'Zurilla, T. J., & Nezu, A. (1982). Social problem solving in adults. In P. C. Kendall (Ed.), *Assessment methods for cognitive behavioral interventions* (pp. 197–226). New York: Academic Press.

Ekstrand, M. L., & Coates, T. J. (1990). Maintenance of safer sexual behaviors and predictors of risky sex: The San Francisco Men's Health Study. *American Journal of Public Health, 80*, 973–977.

Ekstrand, M. L., Stall, R. D., Coates, T. J., & McKusick, L. (1990, June). *Risky sex relapse, the next challenge for AIDS prevention programs: The AIDS Behavioral Research Project.* Paper presented at the Sixth International Conference on AIDS, San Francisco.

Emmons, C. J., Joseph, R., Kessler, C., Wortman, C., Montgomery, S., & Ostrow, D. (1986). Psychosocial predictors of behavior change in homosexual men at risk for AIDS. *Health Education Quarterly, 13*, 331–345.

Evans, K. M. (1987). The female AIDS patient. *Health Care for Women International, 8*, 1–7.

Fairweather, G. W. (Ed.). (1980). *The Fairweather Lodge: A twenty-five year retrospective.* San Francisco: Jossey-Bass.

Fairweather, G. W., Sanders, D. H., & Tornatzky, L. G. (1974). *Creating change in mental health organizations.* New York: Pergamon Press.

Feldman, H. W., & Biernacki, P. (1988). The ethnography of needle sharing among intravenous drug users and implications for public policies and intervention strategies. In R. J. Battjes & R. W. Pickens (Eds.), *Needle sharing among intravenous drug abusers: National and international perspectives.* (NIDA Research Monograph Series No. 80, DHHS Publication No. ADM 88-1567, pp. 28–39). Washington, DC: U.S. Government Printing Office.

Finkel, M. L., & Finkel, D. J. (1975) Sexual and contraceptive knowledge, attitudes, and behavior of male adolescents. *Family Planning Perspective, 7*, 256–260.

Fishbein, M., & Ajzen, I. (1975). *Belief, attitude, intention, and behavior: An introduction to theory and research*. Reading, MA: Addison-Wesley.

Flynn, N. M., Jain, S., Bailey, V., Siegel, B., Banks, V., Nassar, N., Lindo, J., Harper, S., & Ding, D. (1988, June). *Characteristics and stated AIDS risk behavior of IV drug users attending drug treatment programs in a medium-sized U.S. city.* Poster presented at the Fourth International Conference on AIDS, Stockholm.

Fordyce, E. J., Balanon, A., & Stoneburner, R. (1990, June). *Sexual activity among women in the United States and New York City in 1988*. Poster presented at the Sixth International Conference on AIDS, San Francisco.

Friedland, G. H., Harris, C., Small, C. B., Shine, D., Moll, B., Reiss, R., Darrow, W., & Klein, R. (1986). Intravenous drug users and the acquired immune deficiency syndrome (AIDS): Demographic, drug use, and needle sharing patterns. *Archives of Internal Medicine, 145*, 837–840.

Friedman, S. R., de Jong, W. M., & Des Jarlais, D. C. (1988). Problems and dynamics of organizing intravenous drug users for AIDS prevention. *Health Education Research, 3*, 49–57.

Friedman, S. R., & Des Jarlais, D. C. (1989). *Measurement of intravenous drug use behaviors that risk HIV transmission*. Unpublished manuscript, Narcotic and Drug Research, Inc., New York.

Friedman, S. R., Des Jarlais, D. C., Sotheran, J. L., Garber, J., Cohen, H., & Smith, D. (1987). AIDS and self-organization among intravenous drug users. *International Journal of the Addictions, 22*, 201–220.

Friedman, S. R., Sufian, M., Neaigus, Stepherson, B., Manthei, D., Des Jarlais, D. C., Jose, B., Curtis, R., Goldsmith, D., & Mota, P. (1990, June). *Organizing IV drug users against AIDS*. Poster presented at the Sixth International Conference on AIDS, San Francisco.

Fullilove, M. T. (1988). Ethnic minority women and AIDS. *Multicultural Inquiry and Research on AIDS, 2*, 4–5.

Fullilove, M. T., Fullilove, R. E., Haynes, K., & Gross, S. A. (1990a). Black women and AIDS prevention: A view toward understanding the gender rules. *Journal of Sex Research, 27(1)*, 47–64.

Fullilove, M. T., Fullilove, R. E., & Morales, E. (1989). Psychoeducation: A tool for AIDS prevention in minority communities. *Journal of Psychotherapy and the Family, 6(12)*, 143–160.

Fullilove, M. T., Weinstein, M., Fullilove, R. E., Crayton, E. J., Goodjoin, R. B., Bowser, B., & Gross, S. (1990b). Race/gender issues in the sexual transmission of AIDS. *AIDS Clinical Review, 3*, 25–61.

Fullilove, R. E., Fullilove, M. T., Bowser B. P., & Gross S. A. (1989, June). *Crack use and risk for AIDS among black adolescents*. Paper presented at the Fifth International Conference on AIDS, Montreal.

Fullilove, R. E., Fullilove, M. T., Bowser, B. P., & Gross, S. A. (1990a). Risk of sexually transmitted disease among black adolescent crack users in Oakland and San Francisco, CA. *Journal of the American Medical Association,*

263, 851–855.

Fullilove, R. E., Golden, E., Bowser, B. P., & Hulley, S. (1990b, June). *Drug use and sexual behaviors in a probability sample of single adults living in "high risk" neighborhoods of San Francisco, CA: The AMEN Study*. Paper presented at the Sixth International Conference on AIDS, San Francisco.

Galea, R. P., Lewis, B., & Baker, L. (1988). A model for implementing AIDS education in a drug abuse treatment setting. *Hospital and Community Psychiatry, 39*, 886–888.

Gawin, F. H. (1988). Chronic neuropharmacology of cocaine: Progress in pharmacotherapy. *Journal of Clinical Psychiatry, 49*(2, Suppl), 11–16.

Gayle, J. A., Selik, R. M., & Chu, S. Y. (1990). Surveillance for AIDS and HIV infection among black and Hispanic children and women of childbearing age, 1981–1989. *Morbidity and Mortality Weekly Report, 39*(SS-3), 23–30.

Gibson, D. R., Choi, K., Catania, J. A., Sorensen, J. L., & Kegeles, S. (1991). *Psychosocial predictors of needle sharing among intravenous drug users*. Manuscript submitted for publication.

Gibson, D. R., Lovelle-Drache, J., Derby, S., Garcia-Soto, M., & Sorensen, J. L. (1989a, June). *Brief counseling to reduce AIDS risk in intravenous drug users: Update*. Paper presented at the Fifth International Conference on AIDS, Montreal.

Gibson, D. R., Wermuth, L., Lovelle-Drache, J., Ham, J., & Sorensen, J. L. (1989b). Brief counseling to reduce AIDS risk in intravenous drug users and their sexual partners: Preliminary results. *Counselling Psychology Quarterly, 2*, 15–19.

Glaser, E. M., Abelson, H. H., & Garrison, K. N. (1983). *Putting knowledge to use: Facilitating the diffusion of knowledge and the implementation of planned change*. San Francisco: Jossey-Bass.

Gold, M. S., Redmond, D., & Kleber, H. (1978). Clonidine blocks acute opiate withdrawal symptoms. *Lancet, ii*, 599602.

Goldstein, M. J., & Yuen, F. (1988). Coping with AIDS: An approach to training and education in a therapeutic community—the Samaritan Village Program. *Journal of Substance Abuse Treatment, 5*, 4550.

Gross, A., & McMullen, P. (1983). Models of the help-seeking process. In B. DePaulo, A. Nadler, & J. Fisher (Eds.). *New directions in help-seeking and receiving* (Vol. 3, pp. 47–70). New York: Academic Press.

Guydish, J., Abramowitz, A., Woods, W., Black, D. M., & Sorensen, J. L. (1990a). Changes in needle sharing behavior among intravenous drug users: San Francisco, 1986 to 88. *American Journal of Public Health, 80*, 995–997.

Guydish, J., Temoshok, L., Dilley, J., & Rinaldi, J. (1990b). Evaluation of a hospital based substance abuse intervention and referral service for HIV affected patients. *General Hospital Psychiatry, 12*, 1–7.

Haefner, D., & Kirscht, J. (1970). Motivational and behavioral effects of modifying health beliefs. *Public Health Reports, 85*, 478–484.

Haley, J. A. (1978). *Problem-solving therapy*. San Francisco: Jossey-Bass.

Hall, S. M., Sorensen, J. L., & Loeb, P. (1988). Development and diffusion of a skill training intervention. In T. G. Baker & D. S. Cannon (Eds.), *Addic-*

tive disorders: Psychological research on assessment and treatment (pp. 180–204). New York: Praeger Scientific.

Harding, W., & Zinberg, N. (1977). The effectiveness of the subculture in developing rituals and sanctions for controlled drug use. In B. du Toit, (Ed.), *Drugs, rituals, and altered states of consciousness* (pp. 111–133). Rotterdam: A. A. Balkema.

Heitzmann, C. A., Sorensen, J. L., Gibson, D. R., Morales, E. R., Costantini, M., Baer, S., & Purnell, S. (1989, March). *AIDS prevention among IV drug abusers: Behavioral changes.* Poster presented at the meeting of the Society of Behavioral Medicine, San Francisco.

Herek, G. M., & Glunt, E. K. (1988). An epidemic of stigma: Public reactions to AIDS. *American Psychologist, 43*, 886–891.

Hopkins, W. (1988). Needle sharing and street behavior in response to AIDS in New York City. In R. J. Battjes & R. W. Pickens (Eds.), *Needle sharing among intravenous drug abusers: National and international perspectives* (NIDA Research Monograph Series No. 80, DHHS Publication No. ADM 88-1567, pp. 18–27). Washington, DC: U.S. Government Printing Office.

House, J. S. (1981). *Stress and social support.* Reading, MA: Addison-Wesley.

Huang, K. H. C., Watters, J. K., & Case, P. (1989, June). *Predicting compliance with HIV risk reduction among heterosexual intravenous drug users: Relative contributions of health beliefs and situational factors.* Paper presented at the Fifth International Conference on AIDS, Montreal.

Hulley, S. B., & Hearst, N. (1989). The worldwide epidemiology and prevention of AIDS. In V. M. Mays, G. W. Albee, & S. F. Schneider (Eds.), *Primary prevention of AIDS: Psychological approaches* (pp. 47–71). Newbury Park, CA: Sage.

Institute for Health Policy Studies. (1990, February). *The HIV epidemic: New and continuing challenges for the public and private sectors.* Paper prepared for Funders Concerned about AIDS and the Council on Foundations, University of California, San Francisco.

Institute of Medicine, National Academy of Sciences. (1989). *The future of public health.* Washington, DC: National Academy Press.

Jackson, J. F., Rotkiewicz, L. G., Quinones, M. A., & Passannante, M. R. (1989). A coupon program for drug treatment and AIDS education. *International Journal of the Addictions, 24*, 1035–1051.

Jain, S., Flynn, N., Bailey, V., Sweha, A., Ding, D., & Sloan, W. (1989, June). *IVDU and AIDS: More resistance to changing their sexual than their needle-sharing practices.* Poster presented at the Fifth International Conference on AIDS, Montreal.

Janis, I. L. (1967). Effect of fear arousal on attitude change: Recent developments in theory and research. In L. Berkowitz (Ed.), *Advances in experimental social psychology* (Vol. 3, pp. 167–222). New York: Academic Press.

Janz, N., & Becker, M. H. (1984). The health belief model: A decade later. *Health Education Quarterly, 11*, 1–47.

Job, R. F. S. (1988). Effective and ineffective use of fear in health promotion campaigns. *American Journal of Public Health, 78*, 163–167.

Johns Hopkins University School of Hygiene and Public Health. (1986). AIDS:

A public health crisis. *Population Reports*, Series L, No. 6, Issues in World Health.

Johnson, R. E., Cone, E. J., Henningfield, J. E., & Fudala, P. J. (1989). Use of buprenorphine in the treatment of opiate addiction. *Clinical Pharmacology and Therapeutics, 46*(3), 335–343.

Joseph, J., Montgomery, S., Emmons, C., Kessler, R., Ostrow, D., Wortman, C., O'Brien, M., & Eshleman, S. (1987). Magnitude determinants of behavioral risk reduction: Longitudinal analysis of a cohort at risk for AIDS. *Psychology and Health, 75*, 73–96.

Kall, K. I., & Olin, R. G. (1990). HIV status and changes in risk behavior among intravenous drug users in Stockholm 1987–1988. *AIDS, 4*, 153–157.

Kaul, B., & Davidow, B. (1981). Drug abuse patterns of patients on methadone maintenance treatment in New York City. *American Journal of Drug and Alcohol Abuse, 8*, 17–25.

Kegeles, S., Catania, J., Coates, T., & Adler, N. (1986, August). *Sexual risk behavior in a heterogeneous sample seeking AIDS antibody testing*. Paper presented at the annual convention of the American Psychological Association, Washington, DC.

Kelly, J. A., St. Lawrence, J. S., Hood, H. V., & Brasfield, T. L. (1989). Behavioral intervention to reduce AIDS risk activities. *Journal of Consulting and Clinical Psychology, 57*, 60–67.

Kelley, P. W., Miller, R. N., Pomerantz, R., Wann, F., Brundage, J. F., & Burke, D. S. (1990). Human immunodeficiency virus seropositivity among members of the active duty U.S. Army, 1985–1989. *American Journal of Public Health, 80*, 405–410.

Khantzian, E. J. (1979). The ego, the self and opiate addiction: Theoretical and treatment considerations. *International Journal of Psycho-Analysis, 5*, 189–198.

Khantzian, E. J., Mack, J., & Schatzberg, A. (1974). Heroin use as an attempt to cope: Clinical observations. *American Journal of Psychiatry, 131*, 160–164.

Kirscht, J. P., & Joseph, J. G. (1989). The health belief model: Some implications for behavior change with reference to homosexual males. In V. M. Mays, G. W. Albee, & S. F. Schneider (Eds.), *Primary prevention of AIDS: Psychological approaches* (pp. 111–129). Newbury Park, CA: Sage.

Kleber, H. D. (1985). Naltrexone. *Journal of Substance Abuse Treatment, 2*, 117–122.

Kosten, T. R., Morgan, C., & Kleber, H. D. (1990). Buprenorphine treatment of cocaine abuse. *In L. S. Harris (Ed.), Problems of drug dependence, 1989 (NIDA Research Monograph Series* No. 95, DHHS Publication No. ADM 90-1663, p. 461). Washington, DC: U.S. Government Printing Office. (Abstract)

Kosten, T. R., Rounsaville, B. J., & Kleber, H. D. (1987). A 2.5-year follow-up of cocaine use among treated opioid addicts. *Archives of General Psychiatry, 44*, 281–284.

Kroliczak, A. (1990). Update on high-risk behaviors among female sexual partners of injection drug users. *Network, 1*(4), pp. 4–7.

Landesman, S., Minkoff, H., Holman, S., McCalla, S., & Sijin, O. (1987). Serosurvey of human immunodeficiency virus infection in parturients. *Journal of the American Medical Association, 258*, 2701–2703.

Lange, W. R., Snyder, F. R., Lozovsky, D., Kaistha, V., Kaczaniuk, M. A., Jaffee, J. H., & The ARC Epidemiology Collaborating Group. (1988). Geographic distribution of human immunodeficiency virus markers in parenteral drug abusers. *American Journal of Public Health, 78*, 443–446.

Lawson, G. W. (1984). Group counseling in the treatment of chemical dependency. In G. W. Lawson, D. C. Ellis, & P. C. Rivers (Eds.), *Essentials of chemical dependency counseling* (pp. 121–144). Rockville, MD: Aspen.

Leventhal, H., Zimmerman, R., & Gutmann, M. (1984). Compliance: A self-regulation perspective. In W. D. Gentry (Ed.), *Handbook of behavioral medicine* (pp. 369–436). New York: Guilford Press.

Lewis, D. K., & Watters, J. K. (1988). HIV seropositivity and IVDU comparisons [Letter]. *American Journal of Public Health, 78*, 14–99.

Lewis, D. K., & Watters, J. K. (1990, June). *Sexual behavior and sexual self identity in male bisexual and heterosexual IV drug users.* Poster presented at the Sixth International Conference on AIDS, San Francisco.

Lewis, D. K., & Watters, J. K. (1990). *Sexual risk behavior among heterosexual intravenous drug users: Ethnic and gender variations.* Unpublished manuscript.

Lewis, D. K., Watters, J. K., & Case, P. (1990). The prevalence of high-risk sexual behavior in male intravenous drug users with steady female partners. *American Journal of Public Health, 80*, 465–466.

Lex, B. W. (1990). Male heroin addicts and their female mates: Impact on disorder and recovery. *Journal of Substance Abuse, 2*, 147–175.

Lorion, R. P. (1990). Evaluating HIV risk-reduction efforts: Ten lessons from psychotherapy and prevention outcome strategies. *Journal of Community Psychology, 18*, 325–336.

Lowe, D., Milechman, B., Cotton, R., Vumbaca, G., McDermott, R., & Ward, S. (1990, June). *Maximizing return rates and safe disposal of injection equipment in Australian needle syringe exchange programs.* Poster presented at the Sixth International Conference on AIDS, San Francisco.

Lui, K.-J., Darrow, W. W., & Rutherford, G. W. (1988). A model-based estimate of the mean incubation period for AIDS in homosexual men. *Science, 240,* 1333–1335.

Luker, K. (1975). *Taking chances: Abortion and the decision not to contracept.* Berkeley: University of California Press.

MacGregor, R. R. (1987). Alcohol and drugs as co-factors for AIDS. *Advances in Alcohol and Substance Abuse, 7*, 47–71.

Magura, S., Grossman, J. I., Lipton, D. S., Amann, K. R., Koger, J., & Gehan, K. (1989a). Correlates of participation in AIDS education and HIV antibody testing by methadone patients. *Public Health Reports, 104*, 231–240.

Magura, S., Grossman, J. I., Lipton, D. S., Siddiqi, Q., Shapiro, J. L., Marion, I., & Amann, K. R. (1989b). Determinants of needle sharing among intravenous drug users. *American Journal of Public Health, 79*, 459–462.

Magura, S., Shapiro, J. L., Grossman, J. I., & Lipton, D. S. (1989c). Education/

support groups for AIDS prevention with at-risk clients. *Social Casework*, 10–20.

Magura, S., Shapiro, J. L., Siddiqi, Q., & Lipton, D. S. (1990). Variables influencing condom use among intravenous drug users. *American Journal of Public Health, 80*, 82–84.

Magura, S., Siddiqi, Q., Shapiro, J. L., Grossman, J. I., Lipton, D. S., Mario, I. J., Weisenfeld, L., Amann, K. R., & Koger, J. (in press). Outcomes of an AIDS prevention program for methadone patients. *International Journal of the Addictions.*

Margolis, E., Catanzarite, L., Biernacki, P., & Feldman, H. W. (1990, June). *Predictors of safe needle use among intravenous drug users.* In *Proceedings of the Sixth International Conference on AIDS*, San Francisco, Abstract 3025.

Marin, B. V., & Marin, G. (1990, June). *Acculturation differences in Hispanic condom use.* Paper presented at the Sixth International Conference on AIDS, San Francisco.

Marlatt, G. A., & George, W. H. (in press). Relapse prevention and the maintenance of optimal health behavior. In S. Shumaker, E. Schron, & J. K. Ochene (Eds.), *The adoption and maintenance of behaviors for optimal health.* New York: Springer.

Marlatt, G. A., & Gordon, J. R. (Eds.). (1985). *Relapse prevention: Maintenance strategies in the treatment of addiction behaviors.* New York: Guilford Press.

Marlink, R. G., Foss, B., Swift, R., Davis, W., Essex, M., & Groopman, J. (1987, June). *High rates of HTLV-III/LAV exposure in IVDAs from a small city and the failure of specialized methadone maintenance to prevent further drug use.* Paper presented at the Third International Conference on AIDS, Washington, DC.

Marmor, M., Des Jarlais, D. C., Cohen, H., Friedman, S. R., Beatrice, S. T., Dubin, N., El-Sadr, W., Mildvan, D., Yancovits, S., Mathur, U., & Holzman, R. (1987). Risk factors for infection with human immunodeficiency virus among intravenous drug abusers in New York City. *AIDS, 1*, 39–44.

Marmor, M., Des Jarlais, D. C., Friedman, S. R., Lyden, M., & El-Sadr, W. (1984). The epidemic of acquired immunodeficiency syndrome and suggestions for its control in drug abusers. *Journal of Substance Abuse Treatment, 1*, 237–247.

Marvin, S. B., & Steinmetz, S. K. (Eds.). (1987). *Handbook of marriage and the family.* New York: Plenum.

Mata, A. G., Jr., & Jorquez, J. S. (1989). Mexican-American intravenous drug users' needle-sharing practices: Implications for AIDS prevention. In V. M. Mays, G. W. Albee, & S. F. Schneider (Eds.), *Primary prevention of AIDS: Psychological approaches* (pp. 329–344). Newbury Park, CA: Sage.

May, R. M., & Anderson, R. M. (1987). Transmission dynamics of HIV infection. *Nature, 326*, 137–142.

Mays, V. M. (1989). AIDS prevention in black populations: Methods of a safer kind. In V. M. Mays, G. W. Albee, & S. F. Schneider (Eds.), *Primary prevention of AIDS: Psychological approaches* (pp. 264–279). Newbury Park, CA: Sage.

Mays, V. M., & Cochran, S. D. (1988). Issues in the perception of AIDS risk and risk education activities by black and Hispanic/Latina women. *American Psychologist, 43*, 949–957.

McCarthy, J. J., & Borders, O. T. (1985). Limit setting on drug abuse in methadone maintenance patients. *American Journal of Psychiatry, 142*, 1419–1423.

McCusker, J., Stoddard, A., Zapka, J., Morrison, C. C., Phalen, J., & Lewis, B. F. (1990, October). *Evaluation of alternative AIDS educational interventions for drug abusers in treatment (Project SMART)*. Paper presented at the meeting of the American Public Health Association, New York.

McKusick, L., Coates, T. J., & Morin, S. (1990). Longitudinal predictors of reductions in unprotected anal intercourse: Behaviors among gay men in San Francisco. *American Journal of Public Health, 80*, 978–983.

McKusick, L., Coates, T. J., Wiley, J., Morin, S., & Stall, R. (1987, June). *Prevention of HIV infection among gay and bisexual men: Two longitudinal studies*. Paper presented at the Third International Conference on AIDS, Washington, DC.

McKusick, L., Conant, M. A., & Coates, T. J. (1985a). The AIDS epidemic: A model for developing intervention strategies for reducing high risk behavior in gay men. *Sexually Transmitted Diseases, 12*, 229–234.

McKusick, L., Horstman, W., & Coates, T. J. (1985b). AIDS and the sexual behavior reported by gay men in San Francisco. *American Journal of Public Health, 75*, 493–496.

McLellan, A. T., Luborsky, L., & Woody, G. (1983). Predicting response to alcohol and drug abuse treatments: The role of psychiatric severity. *Archives of General Psychiatry, 40*, 620–625.

Medley, G. F., Anderson, R. M., Cox, D. R., & Billard, L. (1987). Incubation period of AIDS in patients infected via blood transfusion. *Nature, 328*, 719–721.

Melton, G. B., Levine, R. J., Koocher, G. P., Rosenthal, R., & Thompson, W. C. (1988). Community consultation in socially sensitive research: Lessons from clinical trials of treatments for AIDS. *American Psychologist, 43*, 573–581.

Michael, R. T., Laumann, E. O., Gagnon, J. H., & Smith, T. W. (1988). Number of sex partners and potential risk of sexual exposure to human immunodeficiency virus. *Morbidity and Mortality Weekly Report*, 37, 565–568.

Miller, H. G., Turner, C. F., & Moses, L. E. (Eds.). (1990). *AIDS: The second decade*. Washington, DC: National Academy Press.

Millman, J., Samet, S., Shaw, J., & Braden, M. (1990). The dissemination of psychological research [Letter]. *American Psychologist, 45*, 668–669.

Minkoff, H. L., Holman, S., Beller, E., Delke, I., Fishbone, A., & Landesman, S. (1988). Routinely offered prenatal HIV testing. *New England Journal of Medicine, 319*, 1018.

Mondanaro, J. (1987). Strategies for AIDS prevention: Motivating drug dependent women. *Journal of Psychoactive Drugs, 19*, 143–149.

Moore, L., Padian, N., Vranizan, K. M., Brodie, B., & Moss, A. R. (1990,

June). *Sexual partners of intravenous drug users in San Francisco.* Poster presented at the Sixth International Conference on AIDS, San Francisco.

Mosley, J., Kramer, T. H., Cancellieri, F., & Ottomenelli, G. (1988, June). *Survey of condom use in substance abusers.* Poster presented at the Fourth International Conference on AIDS, Stockholm.

Moss, A. R. (1987). AIDS and intravenous drug use: The real heterosexual epidemic. British Medical Journal, 294, 389–390.

Moss, A. R., Bachetti, P., Osmond, D., Meakin, R., Keffelew, A., & Gorter, R. (1989, June). *Seroconversion for HIV in intravenous drug users in San Francisco.* Paper presented at the Fifth International Conference on AIDS, Montreal.

Murphy, D. L. (1987). Heterosexual contacts of intravenous drug abusers: Implications for the next spread of the AIDS epidemic. *Advances in Alcohol and Substance Abuse, 7*, 89–97.

Murphy, J. S. (1988). Women with AIDS: Sexual ethics in an epidemic. In I. B. Corless & M. Pittman-Lindeman (Eds.), *AIDS: Principles, practices, and politics* (pp. 665–679). Washington, DC: Hemisphere.

Murphy, S. (1987). Intravenous drug use and AIDS: Notes on the social economy of needle sharing. *Contemporary Drug Problems*, 425–434.

Nathanson, C., & Becker, M. H. (1986). Family and peer influence on obtaining a method of contraception. *Journal of Marriage and the Family, 48*, 513–525.

Nemoto, T., Brown, L. S., Battjes, R. J., & Siddiqui, N. (1990a, June). *Patterns of cocaine use in relation to HIV infection among intravenous drug users in New York City.* Poster presented at the Sixth International Conference on AIDS, San Francisco.

Nemoto, T., Brown, L. S., Foster, K., & Chu, A. (1990b). Behavioral risk factors of human immunodeficiency virus among intravenous drug users and implications for preventive interventions. *AIDS Education and Prevention,* 2, 116–126.

Newmeyer, J. A. (1988). Why bleach? Development of strategy to combat HIV contagion among San Francisco intravenous drug users. In R. J. Battjes & R. W. Pickens (Eds.), *Needle sharing among intravenous drug abusers: National and international perspectives*, (NIDA Research Monograph Series No. 80, DHHS Publication No. ADM 88-1567, pp. 151–159). Washington, DC: Government Printing Office.

Nichols, H. (1988). Narcotics Anonymous. *Journal of Substance Abuse Treatment, 5*, 195–196.

Nova Research Company (1989, Spring). NIDA's NADR Project. *Network*, pp. 12.

Novick, L. F., Berns, D., Stricof, R., Stevens, R., Pass, K., & Wethers, J. (1989). HIV seroprevalence in newborns in New York State. *Journal of the American Medical Association, 261*, 1745–1750.

Nurco, D. N., Wegner, N., Stephenson, P., Makofsky, A., & Shaffer, J. (1983). *Ex-addicts' self-help groups: Potentials and pitfalls.* New York: Praeger.

Padian, N., Marquis, L., Francis, D. P., Anderson, R. E., Rutherford, G. W., O'Malley, P. M., & Winkelstein, W. (1987). Male-to-female transmission of human immunodeficiency virus. *Journal of the American Medical Association, 258*, 788–790.

Padian, N., Peterson, H., Meakin, R., Brodie, B., Wofsy, C., & Moss, A. (1989, June). *Heterosexual transmission of HIV from intravenous drug users to their sexual partners*. Poster presented at the Fifth International Conference on AIDS, Montreal.

Padian, N., Shiboski, S., & Jewell, N. (1990, June). *The relative efficiency of female-to-male HIV sexual transmission*. Poster presented at the Sixth International Conference on AIDS, San Francisco.

Page, B. P., Chitwood, D. D., Smith, P. C., Kane, N., & McBride, D. C. (1990). Intravenous drug use and HIV infection in Miami. *Medical Anthropology Quarterly, 1*, 155–175.

Panem, S. (1987). *The AIDS bureaucracy*. Cambridge, MA: Harvard University Press.

Pappas, L., Gaulard, J., Winterhalter, S., & Christen, P. (1990, June). *Survey of female sexual partners of male IDU's in preparation for HIV prevention campaign*. Poster presented at the Sixth International Conference on AIDS, San Francisco.

Peterson, J. L., & Bakeman, R. (1989). AIDS and IV drug use among ethnic minorities. *Journal of Drug Issues. 19*, 27–37.

Peterson, J. L., & Marin, G. (1988). Issues in the prevention of AIDS among black and Hispanic men. *American Psychologist, 43*, 871877.

Polit-O'Hara, D., & Kahn, J. (1985). Communication and contraceptive practices in adolescent couples. *Adolescence, 20*, 33–42.

Poma, P. A. (1987). Pregnancy in Hispanic women. *Journal of the National Medical Association, 79*, 929–935.

Powell, D. H. (1973). A pilot study of occasional heroin users. *Archives of General Psychiatry, 28*, 586–594.

Presidential Commission on the Human Immunodeficiency Virus Epidemic. (1988). *Report of the Presidential Commission on the HIV Epidemic*. Washington, DC: U.S. Government Printing Office.

Primm, B. J., Brown, L. S., Gibson, B. S., & Chum, A. (1988, June). *The range of sexual behaviors of intravenous drug abusers*. Poster presented at the Fourth International Conference on AIDS, Stockholm.

Puckett, S. B., & Bye, L. (1987). *The Stop AIDS Project: An interpersonal AIDS prevention program*. San Francisco: The Stop AIDS Project.

Purchase, D., Hagan, H., Des Jarlais, D. C., & Reid, T. (1989, June). *Historical account of the Tacoma syringe exchange*. Poster presented at the Fifth International Conference on AIDS, Montreal.

Quinn, T. C., Cannon, R. O., Glasser, D., Groseclose, S. L., Brathwaite, W. S., Fauci, A. S., & Hook, E. W. (1990). The association of syphilis with risk of human immunodeficiency virus infection in patients attending sexually transmitted disease clinics. *Archives of Internal Medicine, 150*, 1297–1302.

Ralph, N., & Spigner, C. (1986). Contraceptive practices among female heroin addicts. *American Journal of Public Health, 76*, 1016–1017.

Rappaport, J., Seidman, E., & Davidson, W. S. (1979). Demonstration research and manifest v. true adoption: The natural history of a research project designed to divert adolescents from the legal system. In R. F. Munoz, L. R. Snowden, & J. G. Kelly (Eds.), *Social and psychological research in community settings: Designing and conducting programs for social and personal well-being* (pp. 101–144). San Francisco: Jossey-Bass.

Raymond, C. A. (1988a). First needle exchange program approved; other cities await results. *Journal of the American Medical Association, 259*, 1289–1290.

Raymond, C. A. (1988b). Study of IV drug users and AIDS finds differing infection rate, risk behavior. *Journal of the American Medical Association, 260*, 3105.

Resnick, L., Veren, K., Salahuddin, S. Z., Tondreau, S., & Markham, P. D. (1986). Stability and inactivation of HTLVIII/LAV under clinical and laboratory environments. *Journal of the American Medical Association, 255*, 1887–1891.

Richardson, J., Schott, J., McGuigan, K., & Levine, A. (1987). Behavior change among homosexual college students to decrease risk for the acquired immune deficiency syndrome. *Preventive Medicine, 16*, 285–286.

Rigby, K., Brown, M., Anagnostou, P., Ross, M. W., & Rosser, B. R. S. (1989). Shock tactics to counter AIDS: The Australian experience. *Psychology and Health, 3*, 145–150.

Rolfs, R. R., Goldberg, M., & Sharrar, R. G. (1990). Risk factors for syphilis: Cocaine use and prostitution. *American Journal of Public Health, 80*, 853–857.

Rogers, E. (1983). *Diffusion of innovation*. New York: Free Press.

Rogers, R. W. (1975). A protection motivation theory of fear appeals and attitude change. *Journal of Psychology, 91*, 93–114.

Rosenbaum, M. (1981a). Sex roles among deviants: The woman addict. *International Journal of the Addictions, 16*, 859–877.

Rosenbaum, M. (1981b). When drugs come into the picture, love flies out the window: Women addicts' love relationships. *International Journal of the Addictions, 16*, 1197–1206.

Rosenshine, N. (1990). Preventing AIDS among female sexual partners of injection drug users: A unique training curriculum. *Network, 1*(4), 1–3.

Rosenstock, I. M. (1974). The health belief model and preventive health behavior. *Health Education Monographs, 2*, 93–114.

Rothenberg, R., Woefel, M., Stoneburner, R., Milberg, J., Parker, R., & Truman, B. (1987). Survival with the acquired immunodeficiency syndrome. *New England Journal of Medicine, 317*, 1297–1302.

Rounsaville, B. J., Weissman, M. M., Crits-Christoph, K., Wilber, C., & Kleber, H. (1982a). Diagnosis and symptoms of depression in opiate addicts. *Archives of General Psychiatry, 39*, 151–156.

Rounsaville, B. J., Weissman, M. M., Kleber, H., & Wilber, C. (1982b). Heterogeneity of psychiatric disorders in treated opiate addicts. *Archives of General Psychiatry, 39*, 161–166.

Samuels, J. (1990). Can IVDUs comply with conventional HIV care? *AIDS Clinical Care, 2*, 34.

San Francisco AIDS Foundation. (1988). *The adventures of Bleachman* [Brochure]. (Available from San Francisco AIDS Foundation, 25 Van Ness St., P. O. Box 6182, San Francisco, CA 94101)

San Francisco Department of Public Health AIDS Office. (1990). *HIV seroprevalence report*. San Francisco: Author.

Saxon, A. J., & Calsyn, D. (1990, June). *Risk behavior of IV stimulant users*. Poster presented at the Sixth International Conference on AIDS, San Francisco.

Schilling, R. F., El-Bassel, N., Gordon, K., & Nichols, S. (1989a, June). *Reducing HIV transmission among recovering female drug users*. Paper presented at the Fifth International Conference on AIDS, Montreal.

Schilling, R. F., El-Bassel, N., Schnike, S., Botvin, G., Orlandi, M., & Nichols, S. (1989b, June). *Risk behavior and attitudes among recovering IV drug users*. Poster presented at the Fifth International Conference on AIDS, Montreal.

Schilling, R. F., El-Bassel, N., Schinke, S. P., Gordon, K., & Nichols, S. Building skills of recovering female drug users to reduce heterosexual AIDS transmisson. *Public Health Reports, 106,* 297–304.

Schinke, S. P., Gilchrist, L. D., & Small, R. W. (1979). Preventing unwanted pregnancy: A cognitive–behavioral approach. *American Journal of Orthopsychiatry, 49*, 8188.

Schoenbaum, E. E., Hartel, D., & Friedland, G. H. (1990, June). *Crack use predicts incident HIV seroconversion*. Paper presented at the Sixth International Conference on AIDS, San Francisco.

Schouten, J., Thorburn, K., Diamond, M., Kendro, B., Partika, N., Peak, A., & Starbuck, G. (1990, June). *A community based effort to establish legal needle exchange in the state of Hawaii*. Poster presented at the Sixth International Conference on AIDS, San Francisco.

Selik, R. M., Castro, K. G., & Pappaioanou, M. (1988). Racial/ethnic differences in the risk of AIDS in the United States. *American Journal of Public Health, 78*, 1539–1545.

Selwyn, P. A., Feiner, C., Cox, C. P., Lipshutz, C., & Cohen, R. L. (1987). Knowledge about AIDS and high-risk behavior among intravenous drug users in New York City. *AIDS, 1*, 247–254.

Selwyn, P. A., Feingold, A., Iezza, A., Satyadeo, M., Colley, J., Torres, R., & Shaw, J. (1989). Primary care for patients with human immunodeficiency virus (HIV) infection in a methadone maintenance treatment program. *Annals of Internal Medicine, 111*, 761–763.

Senay, E. C. (1985). Methadone maintenance treatment. *International Journal of the Addictions, 20*, 803–821.

Serraino, D., & Franceschi, S. (1990, June). *Methadone maintenance programs and AIDS in north Italy*. Paper presented at the Sixth International Conference on AIDS, San Francisco.

Shaw, N. S. (1988, Fall). Preventing AIDS among women: The role of community organizing. *Socialist Review, 100*, 67–92.

Sherr, L. (1990). Fear arousal and AIDS: Do shock tactics work? *AIDS, 4*, 361–364.

Siegel, K., & Gibson, W. C. (1988). Barriers to the modification of sexual behavior among heterosexuals at risk for acquired immunodeficiency syndrome. *New York State Journal of Medicine, 88*, 66–70.

Snyder, F. R., Nemeth-Coslett, R., Myers, M., & Young, P. (1990, June). *Risk behaviors of infrequent IV cocaine users.* Poster presented at the Sixth International Conference on AIDS, San Francisco.

Sorensen, J. L., Batki, S. L., Good, P., & Wilkinson, K. (1989a). Methadone maintenance program for AIDS-affected addicts. *Journal of Substance Abuse Treatment, 6*, 87–94.

Sorensen, J. L., Costantini, M. A., & London, J. A. (1989b). Coping with AIDS: Strategies for patients and staff in drug abuse treatment programs. *Journal of Psychoactive Drugs, 21*(4), 435–440.

Sorensen, J. L., Gibson, D. R. (Executive Producers), & Boudreaux, R. (Producer/Director). (1988a). *Conversations about AIDS and drug abuse* [Videotape]. San Francisco: University of California, San Francisco.

Sorensen, J. L., Gibson, D. R., Heitzmann, C., Calvillo, A., Dumontet, R., Morales, E., & Acampora, A. (1989c). Pilot trial of small group AIDS education with IV drug abusers. In L. S. Harris (Ed.), *Problems of drug dependence, 1988*: (NIDA Research Monograph Series No. 90, DHHS Publication No. ADM 89-1605, p. 60). Washington, DC: U.S. Government Printing Office. (Abstract)

Sorensen, J. L., Gibson, D. R., Heitzmann, C., Dumontet, R., & Acampora, A. (1988b, August). *AIDS prevention with drug abusers in residential treatment: Preliminary results.* Paper presented at the annual convention of the American Psychological Association, Atlanta.

Sorensen, J. L., Gibson, D. R., Heitzmann, C., Dumontet, R., Costantini, M., Melese-d'Hospital, I., London, J., Hulley, S. B., Acampora, A., & Choi, K. H. (1989d, June). *Psychoeducational group approach to AIDS prevention with drug abusers in residential treatment: Impact 6 months after intervention.* Poster presented at the Fifth International Conference on AIDS, Montreal.

Sorensen, J. L., Gibson, D. R., Heitzmann, C., Dumontet, R., & Morales, E. (1989e, August). *AIDS prevention: Behavioral outcomes with outpatient drug abusers.* Poster presented at the annual convention of the American Psychological Association, New Orleans.

Sorensen, J. L., Guydish, J. R., Costantini, M., & Batki, S. (1989f). Changes in needle sharing and syringe cleaning among San Francisco drug abusers [Letter]. *New England Journal of Medicine, 320*, 807.

Sorensen, J. L., Hall, S. M., Loeb, P., Allen, T., Glaser, E. M., & Greenberg, P. D. (1988c). Dissemination of a job seekers' workshop to drug treatment programs. *Behavior Therapy, 19*, 143–155.

Sorensen, J. L., Heitzmann, C., & Guydish, J. R. (1990). Community psychology, drug use, and AIDS. *Journal of Community Psychology, 18*, 347–353.

Sotheran, J. L., Friedman, S. R., Des Jarlais, D. C., Engel, S. D., Weber, J., & Rockwell, R. (1989, June). *Condom use among heterosexual male IV drug users is affected by the nature of social relationships.* Poster presented at the Fifth International Conference on AIDS, Montreal.

Spencer, B. D. (1989). On the accuracy of estimates of numbers of intravenous drug users. In C. F. Turner, H. G. Miller, & L. E. Moses (Eds.), *AIDS: Sexual behavior and intravenous drug use* (pp. 429–446). Washington, DC: National Academy Press.

Stall, R. D., Ekstrand, M., Pollack, L., & Coates, T. J. (1990a, June). *Relapse from safer sex: The AIDS Behavioral Research Project.* Poster presented at the Sixth International Conference on AIDS, San Francisco.

Stall, R. D., Ekstrand, M., Pollack, L., McKusick, L., & Coates, T. J. (1990b). Relapse from safer sex: The next challenge for AIDS prevention efforts. *Journal of Acquired Immune Deficiency Syndrome, 3*, 1181–1187.

Stall, R. D., McKusick, L., Wiley, J., Coates, T. J., & Ostrow, D. G. (1986) Alcohol and drug use during sexual activity and compliance with safe sex guidelines for AIDS: The AIDS Behavioral Research Project. *Health Education Quarterly, 13*, 359–371.

Stall, R. D., & Ostrow, D. (1989). Intravenous drug use, the combination of drugs and sexual activity, and HIV infection among gay and bisexual men: The San Francisco Men's Health Study. *Journal of Drug Issues, 19*(1), 57–75.

Stein, Z. A. (1990). HIV prevention: The need for methods women can use. *American Journal of Public Health, 80*, 460–462.

Stevens, W. F., & Tornatzky, L. G. (1980). The dissemination of evaluation: An experiment. *Evaluation Review, 4*, 339–354.

Stimson, G. V., Alldritt, L., Dolan, K., & Donoghoe, M. (1988). Syringe-exchange schemes for drug users in England and Scotland. *British Medical Journal, 296*, 1717–1719.

Stimson, G. V., & Lart, R. (1990, June). *National survey of syringe-exchanges in England.* Poster presented at the Sixth International Conference on AIDS, San Francisco.

Stone, A. J., Morisky, D., Detels, R., & Braxton, H. (1989). Designing interventions to prevent HIV-1 infection by promoting condoms and spermicides among intravenous drug abusers and their sexual partners. *AIDS Education and Prevention, 1*, 171–183.

Stone, G., Cohen, F., & Adler, N. (1979). *Health psychology.* San Francisco: Jossey-Bass.

Strecher, V., DeVellis, B., Becker, M., & Rosenstock, I. (1986). The role of self-efficacy in achieving health behavior change. *Health Education Quarterly, 13*, 73–91.

Strug, D. L., Hunt, D. E., Goldsmith, D. S., Lipton, D. S., & Spunt, B. (1985). Patterns of cocaine use among methadone clients. *International Journal of the Addictions, 20*, 1163–1175.

Supnick, J. A., & Coletti, G. (1984). Relapse coping and problem solving training following treatment for smoking. *Addictive Behaviors, 9*, 401–404.

Tacconi, F., Edo, S., Gola, T., Lopez, S., Comolli, G., & Giorgio, B. (1990, June). *Heterosexual transmission of HIV: Follow-up (1986–1989) of 142 couples.* Poster presented at the Sixth International Conference on AIDS, San Francisco.

Tennant, F. S., & Sagherian, A. (1987). Double-blind comparison of amantadine and bromocriptine for ambulatory withdrawal from cocaine dependence. *Archives of Internal Medicine, 147*, 109–112.

Tornatzky, L. G., Fergus, E. O., Avellar, J. W., & Fairweather, G. W. (1980). *Innovation and social process*. New York: Pergamon Press.

Treichler, P. A. (1988). AIDS, gender, and biomedical discourse: Current contests for meaning. In E. F. Fee & D. M. Fox (Eds.), *AIDS: The burdens of history* (pp. 190–266). Berkeley: University of California Press.

Turner, C. F., Miller, H. G., & Moses, L. E. (Eds.). (1989). *AIDS: Sexual behavior and intravenous drug use*. Washington, DC: National Academy Press.

U.S. General Accounting Office. (1990). *Methadone maintenance: Some treatment programs are not effective; greater federal oversight needed*. Report to the Chairman, Select Committee on Narcotics Abuse and Control, House of Representatives.

U.S. Senate Committee on the Judiciary. (1990). *Hard-core cocaine addicts: Meeting—and fighting—the epidemic* (Committee Print No. 101.6). Washington, DC: U.S. Government Printing Office.

Valdiserri, R. O. (1989). *Preventing AIDS: The design of effective programs*. New Brunswick, NJ: Rutgers University Press.

Valdiserri, R. O., Arena, V. C., Proctor, D., & Bonati, F. A. (1989). The relationship between women's attitudes about condoms and their use: Implications for condom promotion programs. *American Journal of Public Health, 79*, 499–501.

Van den Hoek, A., & van Haastrecht, H. J. A. (1990, June). *Little change in sexual behavior in drug users in Amsterdam*. Poster presented at the Sixth International Conference on AIDS, San Francisco.

Watters, J. K. (1987). A street-based outreach model of AIDS prevention for intravenous drug users: Preliminary evaluation. *Contemporary Drug Problems, 14*, 411–423.

Watters, J. K. (1988). Meaning and context: The social facts of intravenous drug use and HIV transmission in the inner city. *Journal of Psychoactive Drugs, 20*, 173–177.

Watters, J. K. (1989). Observations on the importance of social context in HIV transmission among intravenous drug users. *Journal of Drug Issues, 19*, 9–26.

Watters, J. K., & Cheng, Y. T. (1987). HIV-1 infection and risk among intravenous drug users in San Francisco: Preliminary results and implications. *Contemporary Drug Problems, 14*, 397–410.

Watters, J. K., Cheng, Y. T., Segal, M., Lorvick, J., Case, P., & Carlson, J. (1990, June). *Epidemiology and prevention of HIV in intravenous drug users in San Francisco, 1986–1989*. Poster presented at the Sixth International Conference on AIDS, San Francisco.

Weber, J., Dengelegi, L., Torquato, S., Kolakathis, A., & Yancovitz, S. (1989, June). *The effects of AIDS education on the knowledge and attitudes toward AIDS by substance abusers in a drug detoxification setting*. Poster presented at the Fifth International Conference on AIDS, Montreal.

Weinstein, N. D. (1980). Unrealistic optimism about future life events. *Journal of Personality and Social Psychology, 39*, 806–820.

Weinstein, N. D. (1982). Unrealistic optimism about susceptibility to health problems. *Journal of Behavioral Medicine, 5*, 441–460.

Weinstein, N. D. (1987, October). *Perceptions of risk*. Paper presented at the Centers for Disease Control Conference on Behavioral Aspects of High Risk Sexual Behavior, Atlanta.

Weisfuse, I. B., Back, S., & O'Hare, D. (1988, June) *The seroprevalence of HIV-1 infection among women attending maternal infant care (MIC) clinics in New York City (NYC)*. Poster presented at the Fourth International Conference on AIDS, Stockholm.

Weiss, S. (1989). Links between cocaine and retroviral infection. *Journal of the American Medical Association, 261*, 607–609.

Weissman, G., Sowder, B., & Young, P. (1990, June). *The relationship between crack cocaine use and other risk factors among women in a national AIDS prevention program—U.S., Puerto Rico, and Mexico*. Paper presented at the Sixth International Conference on AIDS, San Francisco.

Wermuth, L., Choi, K.-H., Ham, J., Falcone, H., & Hulley, S. (1991). *Perceptions of AIDS risk among women sexual partners of injection drug users.* Unpublished manuscript. California State University, Department of Sociology and Social Work, Chico, CA.

Wermuth, L., Falcone, H., & Sorensen, J. (1990, June). *HIV antibody testing in women sexual partners of IVDU*. Poster presented at the Sixth International Conference on AIDS, San Francisco.

Wermuth, L., Ham, J., & Hester, G. (1989, March). *The role of partner cooperation in safer sex*. Poster presented at the meeting of the Society of Behavioral Medicine, San Francisco.

Wermuth, L., Ham, J., & Robbins, R. L. (1991) Women don't wear condoms: AIDS risk among sexual partners of IV drug users. In J. Huber & B. E. Schneider (Eds.), *Social relations and the AIDS crises*. Newbury Park, CA: Sage.

Wiebel, W., Guydan, C., & Chene, D. (1990, June). *Cocaine injection as a predictor of HIV risk behaviors*. Poster presented at the Sixth International Conference on AIDS, San Francisco.

Williams, A., Vranizon, K., Gorter, R., Brodie, B., Meakin, R., & Moss, A. (1990, June). *Methadone maintenance, HIV serostatus and race in injection drug users (IDU) in San Francisco, CA*. Poster presented at the Sixth International Conference on AIDS, San Francisco.

Williams, M. L. (1990). HIV seroprevalence among male IVDUs in Houston, Texas. *American Journal of Public Health, 80*, 1507–1508.

Winkelstein, W., Wiley, J., Padian, N., Samuel, M., Shiboski, S., Ascher, M., & Levy, J. (1988). The San Francisco Men's Health Study: Continued decline in HIV seroconversion rates among homosexual/bisexual men. *American Journal of Public Health, 78*, 1472–1474.

Wofsy, C. B. (1987, April). *Intravenous drug abuse and women's medical issues*. Report of the Surgeon General's workshop on children with HIV infection and their families (pp. 32–34). Washington, DC: United States Department of Health/Public Service.

Wolfe, H., Vranizan, K. M., Gorter, R. G., Cohen, J. B., & Moss, A. R. (1990, June). *Crack use and related risk factors in IVDUs in San Francisco.* Poster presented at the Sixth International Conference on AIDS, San Francisco.

Wolk, J., Wodak, A., Morlet, A., Guinan, J. J., Wilson, E., Gold, J., & Cooper, D. A. (1988). Syringe HIV seroprevalence and behavioral and demographic characteristics of intravenous drug users in Sydney, Australia, 1987. *AIDS, 2*, 373–377.

Worth, D. (1989). Sexual decision-making and AIDS: Why condom promotion among vulnerable women is likely to fail. *Studies in Family Planning, 20*, 297–307.

Worth, D., & Rodriguez, R. (1987, Jan.–Feb.). Latina women and AIDS. *SIECUS Report*, pp. 5–7.

Wurtele, S., & Maddux, J. (1987). Relative contributions of protection motivation theory components in predicting exercise intentions and behavior. *Health Psychology, 6*, 453–466.

Yalom, I. D. (1985). *Theory and practice of group psychotherapy.* New York: Basic Books.

Yano, E. M., Gorman, E. M., Kanouse, D. E., Berry, S. H., & Abrahamse, A. (1990, June). *The epidemiology of risk behavior in Los Angeles: Population-based comparison of gay/bisexual men and the general population.* Poster presented at the Sixth International Conference on AIDS, San Francisco.

Young, P., Snyder, F., Friedman, S., & Myers, M. (1990, June). *Racial and geographic differences in risk behaviors of intravenous drug users.* Paper presented at the Sixth International Conference on AIDS, San Francisco.

Zagury, D., Bernard, J., Leonard, R., Cheynier, R., Feldman, M., Sarin, P., & Gallo, R. (1986). Long-term cultures of HTLV-III-infected T-cells: A model of cytopathology of T-cell depletion in AIDS. *Science, 231*, 850–853.

Zahn, M. A., & Ball, J. C. (1974). Patterns and causes of drug addiction among Puerto Rican females. *Addictive Diseases, 1*, 203–213.

Appendix: Where to Get Help or Information

LINDA E. RICO

INTRODUCTION: HOW TO USE THIS APPENDIX

This appendix explains how to find the help or information necessary to prevent AIDS in drug users and their sexual partners. It is divided into three categories: "Organizations," "Information," and "Further Reading or Other Media Sources." "Organizations" lists national or international membership groups created to address specific concerns. Under "Information" are listed resources for education. *"Further Reading or Other Media Sources"* include books and other publications, and additional media sources such as films and videos. Within each category are sections pertaining to AIDS, drug abuse, and issues related to sexual partners, when available. Resources are listed in alphabetical order for easy access. The listing of a particular resource does not qualify as an endorsement; rather, it is intended solely for assistance in obtaining more information on AIDS and drug abuse issues.

ORGANIZATIONS

Organizations of AIDS Agencies

ACT UP Network
P.O. Box 190712
Dallas, TX 75219
(816) 753-3505

This is a national network of AIDS activist groups. They work for funding of AIDS education and services, and for the release of treatments for AIDS.

Association of Asian Pacific Community Health Organizations
1212 Broadway, 730

Oakland, CA 94612
(415) 272-9536

This organization provides technical support to its 8 member clinics in the areas of advocacy, health promotion, and uniforming patient demographic and clinical data. It also has a health education video developed for Asian/Pacific Islander populations available in English, Cantonese, Korean, Samoan, Tagalog, Vietnamese, and Laotian.

National Association of People with AIDS
2025 I St., N.W., Suite 415
Washington, DC 20006
(202) 429-2856

Organized by and for people with AIDS, this is a network of local groups that advocates for people with AIDS.

National Coalition of Black Lesbians and Gays
19641 West Seven Mile
Detroit, MI 48219
(313) 537-0484

A network of local groups that provides speakers and workshop leaders, as well as a training manual for AIDS educators.

National Coalition of Hispanic Health and Human Services Organizations (COSSMHO)
1030 15th St., N.W., Suite 1053
Washington, DC 20005
(202) 371-2100

This is a coalition of organizations and individuals involved in policy, research, national demonstrations, and materials development in the areas of AIDS, chronic diseases, alcohol and substance abuse, maternal and child health, mental health, and social services.

National Lawyers Guild AIDS Network
558 Capp St.
San Francisco, CA 94110
(415) 824-8884

This group of advocates addresses issues of AIDS, public policy, and the law. Services include a practice manual, quarterly newsletter, and national legal referrals.

Organizations Related to Drug Use

Alcohol, Tobacco and Other Drugs Section
American Public Health Association
1015 15th St., N.W.
Washington, DC 20005
(202) 789-5600

This organization, devoted to the protection and promotion of public health, publishes materials on the latest findings in drug abuse treatment and research.

International Working Group on AIDS and Drug Use
Narcotic and Drug Research, Inc.
11 Beach St.
New York, NY 10013
(212) 966-8700

This group provides information on AIDS and drug use through enhancing research and publication of a newsletter.

Society of Psychologists in Addictive Behaviors
President Raymond F. Hanbury, PhD
JFK Johnson Rehabilitation Institute
Edison, NJ 08818
and
Mount Sinai School of Medicine
New York, NY 10003
(908) 321-7721

This organization of psychologists working with addiction publishes a quarterly journal to encourage communication among professionals in this field.

INFORMATION

Information about AIDS

American Foundation for AIDS Research
5900 Wilshire Blvd., 2nd floor East
Los Angeles, CA 90036-5032
(212) 719-0033

This group is the source for the *AIDS Information Resources Directory,* and a major funder of research and public service grants to prevent or treat AIDS.

Multicultural Prevention Resources Corporation
1540 Market St., Suite 320
San Francisco, CA 94102
(415) 861-2142

This group assists in AIDS educational training for people of color.

National AIDS Hotline
(800) 342-AIDS

This provides 24-hour, 7-day-a-week information and referrals about AIDS.

National AIDS Clearinghouse (NAC)
P.O. Box 6003
Rockville, MD 20849-6003
(800) 458-5231

The NAC is the Centers for Disease Control's primary reference, referral, and publications distribution service for HIV and AIDS information. The Clearinghouse acquires, organizes, reviews, updates, and distributes this information.

National Center for Health Education
72 Spring St.
New York, N.Y. 10012
(212) 689-1886

This organization offers a comprehensive health education curriculum for primary schools that includes lessons on AIDS in grades K–6. The curriculum is now used by 8,000 schools in 45 states.

National Hemophilia Foundation
110 Greene St., Room 406
New York, NY 10012
(212) 219-8180
(800) 424-2634 (information center)

This organization offers publications, provides workshops and advocacy, and is involved in research on hemophilia and AIDS. The information center focuses on hemophilia and HIV.

National Institute on Justice
AIDS Clearinghouse
National Criminal Justice Reference Service
P.O. Box 6000
Rockville, MD 20850
(800) 851-3420

The clearinghouse will answer questions, make referrals, and suggest pertinent publications on AIDS and criminal justice issues, such as policies and procedures for law enforcement and corrections agencies.

National Minority AIDS Council
714 G St. SE
P.O. Box 28574
Washington, DC 20003
(202) 544-1076

This group helps communities to develop volunteer programs, provides training and technical expertise, supplies publications and referrals, and advocates on behalf of minorities.

National Native American AIDS Prevention Center
3515 Grand Ave., Suite 100
Oakland, CA 94610
(415) 444-2051
(800) 283-2437 National Indian AIDS Line

NNAAPC provides training, technical assistance, and information services to American Indian/Alaskan Native/Native Hawaiian communities throughout the U.S. It also sponsors the National Indian AIDS Media Consortium.

National Resource Center on Women and AIDS
Center for Women Policy Studies
2000 P St. NW, Suite 508
Washington, DC 20036
(202) 872-1770

This organization produces annually *The Guide to Resources on Women and AIDS*. It also produces policy papers on women and AIDS issues, works on federal policy change, and has produced a video, *Fighting for Our Lives: Women Confronting AIDS*.

National Women's Health Network
1325 G St. NW, Lower Level
Washington, DC 20005
(202) 347-1140

This group publishes educational materials for women about AIDS.

Office of HIV/AIDS Education
American Red Cross
1709 New York Ave. NW, #208
Washington, DC 20006
(202) 639-3223

This agency supplies HIV/AIDS education, training opportunities, and materials. Specific programs for Hispanic and African-American communities are available.

Project Inform
347 Dolores St., Suite 301
San Francisco, CA 94110
(415) 558-9051

This organization provides information on drug therapies for HIV infection, including alternative treatments and approved drugs.

Information about Drug Abuse

Association for Drug Abuse Prevention and Treatment (ADAPT)
302 Bedford Avenue

Brooklyn, NY 11201
(718) 782-2080

This is an organization of addicts in recovery who provide education and training for prevention of AIDS among injection drug users.

National Clearinghouse for Alcohol and Drug Abuse Information (NCADI)
P.O. Box 2345
Rockville, MD 20852
(800) 729-2600

The NCADI provides information and services to anyone with any questions or concerns about any kind of drug problem. It also provides publications, films, videos, references, and referrals.

Information about Sexual Partner Issues

California Prostitutes Education Project—Oakland
811 Clay Street
Oakland, CA 94607

California Prostitutes Education Project—San Francisco
333 Valencia Street, Suite 101
San Francisco, CA 94103

A non-profit AIDS/HIV education and prevention organization, serving four Bay Area Counties; Alameda, San Francisco, Marin, and Contra Costa. Target populations served: sex workers and their regular sexual partners; injection drug users and their regular sexual partners; women who engage in high-risk sexual behavior; juveniles (incarcerated); and adult offenders (incarcerated). The Vocational Reorientation Program assists women who want to change professions. "Each one Teach one" is the motto of CAL-PEP.

Education Department
Planned Parenthood Federation of America
810 Seventh Ave.
New York, NY 10019
(212) 603-4626

This department acts as a clearinghouse with data bases on sexuality and AIDS, education materials, publications, and films.

Haitian Women's Program
American Friends Service Committee
15 Rutherford Place
New York, NY 10003
(212) 598-0965

This program provides AIDS education and prevention information for Haitians.

Project AWARE (Association for Women's AIDS Research and Education)
San Francisco General Hospital Ward 95
1001 Potrero Ave.
San Francisco, CA 94110
(415) 476-4091

This is a University of California-funded research project examining the risk of AIDS for women in San Francisco.

Sex Information and Education Council of the United States (SIECUS)
32 Washington Place
New York, NY 10003
(212) 673-3850

This organization offers a resource bank on AIDS education, as well as a speakers' bureau.

Women's AIDS Network
c/o San Francisco AIDS Foundation
P.O. Box 6182
San Francisco, CA 94101-6182
(415) 864-4376 Ext. 2007

This agency acts as a source of information exchange, support, and assistance to its members, and develops ways to direct HIV/AIDS services and education to women with HIV/AIDS.

Women and AIDS Resource Network (WARN)
30 Third Avenue, Suite 212
Brooklyn, NY 11217
(718) 596-6007

Women can receive information, publications, support, and advocacy concerning AIDS issues from this organization.

FURTHER READING OR OTHER MEDIA SOURCES

Publications on AIDS

Newsletters

AIDS Clinical Care
1440 Main St.
Waltham, MA 02154-1649

AIDS Treatment News
John S. James, Publisher

P.O. Box 411256
San Francisco, CA 94141

BETA (Bulletin of Experimental Treatments for AIDS)
San Francisco AIDS Foundation
P.O. Box 2189
Berkeley, CA 94702-0189

Focus: A Guide to AIDS Research and Counseling
P.O. Box 0884
San Francisco, CA 94143-0884

MIRA (Multicultural Inquiry and Research on AIDS)
Bayview–Hunter's Point Foundation
5815 Third St.
San Francisco, CA 94124

BOOKS

Calen, M. (Ed.). (1987–1988). *Surviving and Thriving with AIDS: Hints for the Newly Diagnosed* (2 vols.). New York: People with AIDS Coalition, Inc.

Delaney, M., & Goldblum, P. (1987). *Strategies for Survival: A Gay Men's Health Manual for the Age of AIDS.* New York: St. Martin's Press.

Lambda Legal Defense and Education Fund. (1987). *Living with AIDS: A Guide to the Legal Problems of People with AIDS.* New York: Author.

Martelli, L. (1987). *When Someone You Know Has AIDS: A Practical Guide.* New York: Crown.

Moffat, B., & Spiegel, J. (1987). *AIDS: A Self-Care Manual.* Los Angeles: AIDS Project Los Angeles.

VIDEOTAPES

Conversations About AIDS and Drug Abuse
Produced by Saccade Communications
Substance Abuse Services, Ward 92
San Francisco General Hospital
1001 Potrero Avenue
San Francisco, CA 94110

This film intends to generate discussion about AIDS and drug use. It is a videotape of drug abusers, many of whom have contracted AIDS—interviews that allow them to tell their stories. The tape proceeds in brief segments, which can stimulate discussion of several issues concerning AIDS and drug abuse. In the segments, the participants discuss the threat of

AIDS and how they learned that they were affected by it, risk factors for HIV infection, their identity as drug users, barriers to lowering the risk of sexual transmission, the problem of denial, and the changes needed in the drug-using community.

Publications on Drug Use

Newsletters

ADAMHA News
Alcohol, Drug Abuse, and Mental Health Aministration
Room 13C-05
5600 Fishers Lane
Rockville, MD 20857
(301) 443-0746

Newsletter of the International Working Group on AIDS and Drug Use
Narcotic and Drug Research, Inc.
11 Beach St.
New York, NY 10013

NIDA Notes
National Institute on Drug Abuse
Room 10A-54
Rockville, MD 20857

Of Substance
Legal Action Center, Inc.
153 Waverly Place
New York, NY 10014

Books

Galea, R., Lewis, B., & Baker, L. (Eds.). (1988). *AIDS and IV Drug Users.* Owings Mills, MD: Rynd Communications.

Sorensen, J. L., & Bernal, G. (1987). *A Family Like Yours: Breaking the Patterns of Drug Abuse.* San Francisco: Harper & Row.

Sulima, J. (Ed.). (1987) *What Every Drug Counselor Should Know about AIDS.* Washington, DC: Manisses Communicatioins.

Publications on Sexual Partner Issues

Journals

Focus on Women
1315 Walnut St., Suite 905
Philadelphia, PA 19102

BOOKS

Delacorte, F., & Alexander, P. (Eds.). (1987). *Sex Work*. Pittsburgh: Cleis Press.

Everett, J., & Glanz, W. (1987). *The Condom Book: Essential Guide for Men and Women*. New York: New American Library/Signet.

Institute for the Advanced Study of Human Sexuality. (1986). *Safe Sex in the Age of AIDS: Guidelines for Reducing the Risk of Contracting AIDS During Sexual Contact*. Secaucus, NJ: Citadel Press.

Patton, C., & Kelly, J. (1987). *Making It: A Woman's Guide to Sex in the Age of AIDS*. Ithaca, NY: Firebrand Books.

Index

Abstinence, 10, 12, 107, 108, 123
Addiction, 18, 24–25, 56
African-Americans
  and AIDS risk reduction model, 73–74
  and drug use during sex, 56–57
  HIV infection in, 8–9, 31, 32, 34, 44, 45, 169
  and injection drug use, 28, 30–31, 36, 44–45
  media campaign for, 60, 96, 135
  in military, 47–48
  and pediatric AIDS, 169
  and prostitution, 50–51
  women, AIDS risk in, 131, 132, 169
AIDS
  deaths from, 4, 23, 131
  diagnosis of, 4
  distribution of, 44–45
  first recognition of, 4
  information about, 204–206
  medical problems of, 4–5, 81, 88–90
  as moral violation, 18, 59
  organizations, 202–203
  pediatric; *see* Infants
  publications about, 208–210
  regional variation in, 8
  statistics on, 5–6, 9, 12–13, 28, 31, 43, 131
"AIDS Antibody Testing at Alternative Test Sites," 110
"AIDS Rap" song, 113
AIDS risk reduction model (ARRM), 15, 61, 62, 63–67, 72–73, 116–117
  elements of, 64–65, 72
AIDS vaccine, 4
AIDS-related complex (ARC), 81, 120
Alcohol, for needle cleaning, 38, 106, 165
Alcohol use
  and immune suppression, 79
  medications for, 81
  and sexual risk behaviors, 7, 132, 173
Altruism, appeals to, 91, 171, 172
Amphetamines, 7
Anal intercourse, 50, 56, 126, 127
Anger, 92
Antidepressants, 81, 86
Antiparkinsonian drugs, 86
Antisocial behavior, 92
Anxiety, AIDS-specific, 71, 92, 93, 94, 102, 120
  and denial, 21, 22, 71, 148
  and perceived severity of disease, 71, 118
  treatment of, 95
  and use of condoms, 124
  in women sexual partners, 146
Aversive emotions, 64–65
AZT, 4, 83, 89

B

Barrier methods, 12; *see also* Condom use
Beck Depression Inventory, 93
Beck Hopelessness Scale, 93
Behavior change, 62, 126
  and health belief model, 63
  in injection drug users, 28, 35–40, 41, 54

Behavior change (*continued*)
and perception of AIDS risk, 53
relapse in, 39, 42, 56, 70, 114, 126, 177
and self-efficacy, 61, 63, 69, 70
in sexual behavior, 54–56
stages of, 64–65
Benzodiazepines, 81, 95
Bisexuality, 48, 50
Blaming victims, 59
Bleach, for cleaning needles, 106, 165
in case examples, 19, 22
distribution of, 9, 12, 38, 40, 128, 161
as drug paraphernalia, 20
increase in use of, 13, 36, 38, 54
"Bleachman," 41
Brandt, Allan M. (quoted), 18, 168
Buprenorphine, 82, 86–87
Buspirone, 95, 97

C

Central nervous system depressants, 7
Clonidine, 81, 82
Cocaine Anonymous (CA), 79, 173
Cocaine use, 7, 35, 77, 97, 174
antidepressant treatment for, 81, 86, 87
buprenorphine treatment for, 86–87
in case example, 25–26
and HIV infection, 31–32, 34, 42
and immune suppression, 79
and methadone maintenance treatment, 86–87
regional variation in, 8
and risk behavior, 37
Codeine, 19
Codependency, 146
Commitment stage, in AIDS risk reduction model, 64, 65, 72
and self-efficacy, 69, 117
Communication
and condom use, 58–59
and cultural values, 59
lack of, 56
skills, 65, 66, 70, 74, 100–101, 117
Community consultation, 166
Community-based campaigns, 40, 41, 61, 134, 172
importance of in minority communities, 61
Condom use, 12, 19, 132, 144, 145
attitudes toward, 57–58, 141, 146, 178
costs/benefits of, 141–142
by drug injectors, 52–53, 54–56, 70, 169
education for, 102, 106–107, 109, 115, 124–125
failures in, 123
and free distribution, 175
male resistance to, 18, 23, 57–58, 124, 133, 141–142
promotion programs for, 25
and self-efficacy, 70, 102
Contraceptive use, 58, 133
"Conversation about AIDS and Drug Abuse," 108
Coping skills, 92, 129
Counseling, 13, 15, 25, 60, 81, 91, 173
grief, 91
group; *see* Group counseling
individual; *see* Individual counseling
by minority group members, 61
pre/post–HIV antibody testing, 175
for women, 130, 134, 136
Counseling Women about HIV Risk: A Checklist, 138–139
Crack; *see also* Cocaine
and sexual risk behaviors, 7, 32, 132
use of by women, 132

D

Dangle, Lloyd, 120, 121
Daytop Village (New York), 80
Decision-making theory, 62
Dementia, 26, 92, 94
Denial, of risk, 14, 21, 24, 56, 59, 68, 92
and anxiety, 21, 22
by women sexual partners, 145–146, 148

Dependence, economic/emotional, 56, 58, 145, 178
Depression
in HIV-infected patients, 84, 87, 88, 90, 92, 93–94
in women sexual partners, 146
Desipramine, 86
Detoxification programs, 81–82, 102, 103, 122, 173, 174
group education in, 111–112
Dilaudid, 7
Dissemination techniques, 162–163, 164–166
Disulfiram, 81
Dopamine agonists, 86
Drug culture
gender roles in, 30, 133
sharing in, 29–31, 169
socialization to, 29
Drug treatment programs, 77–98, 173–175; *see also* Counseling; Detoxification programs; Methadone maintenance treatment; Residential treatment programs
in clinics, 21, 28–29, 40, 136, 173, 174
couple-oriented approaches in, 60,
educational, 61, 94, 96, 99, 102, 136
medical treatment in, 90–95
mental health treatment in, 90–95
referrals to, 122
training of counselors in, 61
types of, 79–82
Drug-free treatment, 81
Drugs of abuse, 7–8

E

Education, 13, 25, 74, 99, 170–173
about drug abuse, 206–207, 210
in drug treatment centers, 61, 94, 96, 102, 136
on HIV transmission, 96, 204–206
through mass media, 20, 21, 134, 135
in medical clinics, 135
posters, 23, 113
about sexual partner issues, 207–208, 210–211
about sexually transmitted diseases, 174
shock tactics in, 160–161
Enactment stage, in AIDS risk reduction model, 64, 65, 72
and self-efficacy, 70, 117
Ethnic minority populations, 112–113; *see also* African-Americans; Hispanic population; Women, minority
Ethnographic studies, 36, 155–156, 166
Evaluating AIDS Prevention Programs (Coyle et al.), 176

F

Fear, in media campaigns, 160–161, 171
Fluoxetine, 87, 97

G

Grief, 91
Group counseling, 99–115, 128, 147
advantages vs. disadvantages of, 100
and cocaine abuse, 87
education programs in, 15, 20, 23, 101–102, 105–114
elements of, 104
homework in, 104, 108, 109, 111
promoting, 105
tools for, 105–106

H

Halfway houses, 95
Hallucinogens, 8
Health belief model, 60–61, 62, 63, 100–101
and susceptibility, 68

Health care systems, 4, 24
Health psychology, 62, 100
Heroin, 7, 35, 65, 81
  and methadone maintenance treatment, 81, 85
Heterosexual population; *see also* Transmission of HIV, heterosexual
  education of, 136
  HIV infection in, 5–6, 23, 43–49
  and knowledge of AIDS, 67
  neglect of, 23, 24
  seroprevalence in, 45–48
Hispanic population
  condom use in, 59, 60, 133
  HIV infection in, 8–9, 31, 32, 34, 44, 45, 169
  injection drug use in, 28, 31, 45
  media campaigns for, 60, 96, 135
  in military, 47–48
  pediatric AIDS in, 169
  women in, 45, 53, 59, 96, 131, 132, 133
HIV antibody testing, 11, 12, 13, 22, 142–143, 173
  as adjunct to counseling, 126–127, 175
  anonymous, 25, 175
  discussion of in group counseling, 110
  in monogamous relationships, 124
  negative results of, 142
HIV infection, 4; *see also* AIDS
  in case examples, 25–26, 82, 88, 90–91
  defense lines against, 10–12
  early symptoms of, 68
  ethnic/cultural patterns in, 9, 42, 45, 95
  prevalence patterns in, 45–49
  and psychological distress, 84, 92, 94
  regional variation in, 8, 45–47, 169
  stabilization of, 33, 41
  transmission of; *see* Transmission
Homosexual populations, 56, 58, 114–115; *see also* San Francisco, AIDS epidemic in
  AIDS knowledge in, 67
  high-risk behaviors in, 126, 127, 177, 178
  injection drug use in, 96
  prejudice toward, 59
  and response efficacy, 69
  and social support, 71
Hopelessness, 93
How to Get Your Lover to Use a Condom and Why You Should (Breitman et al.), 124
"How People Get AIDS" (cartoon), 120, 121
Human immunodeficiency virus (HIV), 4

I

Immune system, 4, 79
Individual counseling, 20, 21, 22, 116–129
  advantages vs. disadvantages of, 147
  elements of, 117–118
  follow-up, 125–126
  and HIV antibody testing, 126–127
  outcome of in heroin detoxification outpatients, 125
  problem solving in, 118–119, 124, 126, 129, 134, 139
  tools for, 119
  for women, 134, 136–149
Infants, HIV infection in, 23, 43, 45, 46, 47, 130
Infections, secondary, 71, 79, 92
Injection drug use, 6–9, 17*n*, 18, 122
  case examples of, 18–21, 24–25
  "closeted," 24–25
  in homosexual populations, 96
  and immune suppression, 79
  indicators of, 6–7
  patterns of, 6–7, 9, 28, 30–31, 73, 168
  regional variation in, 8, 45–47
  seroprevalence in, 13, 31, 33–34
  sexual behavior in, 49, 50–53, 57, 78

transient lifestyles in, 156
by women, 23, 30, 31, 133
Institute of Medicine, 161
Insurance coverage, discrimination in, 59
Isolation, feelings of, 92, 94

J

Job training liaison, 174

K

Knowledge, of AIDS, 64, 65, 67–68, 117

L

Labeling, 64, 65, 72
Local government, 21
Lubricants, 106, 124–125

M

Machismo, 60
Male role models, 136, 171
Marijuana, 79
Mass media, 20, 21, 60, 134, 135
Material support
for AIDS patients, 26, 94, 174
for women sexual partners, 140
Medical problems concurrent with AIDS, 4–5, 81, 88–90
Mental health services, 91
case management in, 95
levels of, 94–95
Methadone, 25, 81
stopping treatment with, 84
Methadone maintenance treatment (MMT), 77, 78, 81–91, 98, 102, 122
case examples of, 78, 82, 88, 90–91
limit setting in, 84–85
medical treatment in, 88–90
patient statistics, 81
preferential admission in, 84
treatment outcome in, 85
MidCity Consortium to Combat AIDS (San Francisco), 38
Military recruits, HIV infection in, 8, 46, 47
Monogamous relationships, 12, 107, 109, 149, 170
and antibody testing, 124
Mood disorders, 92
Morphine, 7
Moss, Andrew (quoted), 6

N

Naltrexone, 81–82
Narcotics Anonymous (NA), 79, 111, 114, 122, 173
National AIDS Demonstration Research (NADR) Project, 40–41, 52, 147, 169
National Institute on Drug Abuse, 40
National Opinion Research Center, 49
National Research Council, 176
Needle Cleaning and Condom Use Checklist, 106, 123
Needle exchange programs, 9, 10, 20, 25, 40, 41, 176
illegal, 13, 175
Needle sharing, 10, 29–30, 39–40, 42, 62, 72–74, 144, 177
and appeals to altruism, 91
attempts to prevent, 10
in case example, 22
decrease in, 13, 35, 36, 37, 41, 54, 55–56
demographic characteristics of, 66
and economic factors, 66, 73
male–female, 133
among minorities, 31, 32, 66, 73, 169
and self-efficacy, 70, 72
underreporting of, 31, 32

Needles, 14
in case example, 24
cleaning of, 11–12, 38–40, 41, 72, 107, 108, 144, 165
education about, 10–11, 13
exchange of; *see* Needle exchange programs
sales of, 35, 36
and sexual activity, 12, 30
sharing; *see* Needle sharing
Networks
in homosexual populations, 115
importance of, 20, 21
in minority communities, 20, 61
needle-sharing, 31, 169
New York
AIDS epidemic in, 12, 33, 34–35, 42
risk-behavior change in, 35–37, 39, 41

O

Opiates, 7, 79, 81, 82; *see also* Heroin
medication for dependence on, 81–82
Outpatient treatment, 81–82, 88; *see also* Methadone maintenance treatment
group work in, 101–102
medical, 88–90, 97
for women, 101, 136
Outreach programs, 13, 40, 41, 172–173, 175
and distribution of bleach, 38
individual, 20, 22
lack of funds for, 172
of local government, 21
streetwise workers in, 128
for women, 134–136

P

Parenting education, liaison to, 174
Partner notification programs, 174–175
Partners Outreach Project, 59, 137–146
Pentamidine, 83, 89
Phoenix House (New York), 80
Physical abuse, 19, 53, 132, 142
Plans to Reduce Risk form, 119, 122, 123, 124, 126
Police harassment, 20
Posters, 23, 113
Poverty
and AIDS, 9, 130, 132
and mental health problems, 149
Power imbalance, in male–female relationships, 56, 58, 59, 132, 133
Prevention programs
adoption of by policymakers, 154–160, 163–164, 166–167
for AIDS, 101–102, 153–167
assessment of, 156–157, 166
for drug use, 10–12
with ethnic and sexual minorities, 95–96, 112–113
Program for AIDS Counseling and Education (PACE), 83–85
limit setting in, 84–85
Prostitution, 23, 50, 53
use of condoms in, 131
Psychedelics, 8
Psychiatric medications, 26, 81, 94–95, 97
abuse of, 94–95
Psychiatric problems concurrent with AIDS, 91–95
in case example, 90–91
and increased drug use, 91
and treatment outcome, 93
Psychoeducational groups; *see* Group counseling
Psychotherapy, 26, 81, 94, 97

R

Relapse, problem of, 39, 42, 56, 70, 114, 126, 130–132, 177
Relationships
caretaking role in, 146–147

long-term, changes in, 144–145, 146
monogamous, 12, 107, 109, 124, 149, 170
need for equality in, 178
power imbalance in, 56, 58, 59, 132, 133
Research projects, 21, 97–98, 176–178
Residential treatment programs, 80–81, 95, 97, 122
group education in, 102–103, 111
Response efficacy, 64, 66, 68–69, 117, 125
and behavior change, 69
Risk behaviors
analysis of, 61, 64, 114
and behavior change, 28, 35–40, 41, 54–56
denial of, 14, 21, 24, 56, 59, 68
sociological perspective on, 177
Role playing, 109, 117, 124, 128

S

Safe(r) sex, 12, 53, 56, 177; *see also* Condom use
and HIV antibody testing, 127
in monogamous relationships, 124
and prevention programs, 12, 109
San Francisco
AIDS epidemic in, 13, 33–34, 35, 42
gay men in, 56
high-risk groups in, 50, 56, 114, 128
outreach program in, 38
Program for AIDS Counseling and Education (PACE) in, 83
risk-behavior change in, 36, 37–40, 41
San Francisco General Hospital, 3, 65
Substance Abuse Services, 78, 83, 89
San Francisco Men's Health Study, 56
Sedative-hypnotics, 7
Self-assessment tools, 114
Self-efficacy, 62, 63, 64, 66, 69–70, 74, 103
in individual counseling, 117, 125, 128, 147
sex-related, 102
in women, 132, 134
Self-help programs, 26, 60, 79–80, 94, 97, 172, 174
Self-interest, appeals to, 91–92
Self-management skills, 126, 129
Self-report, of drug use, 159–160, 176
Seroconversion rates, 33–35, 41, 42
Sexual activities, 9, 14, 49–50; *see also* Monogamous relationships; Safe(r) sex
avoidance of, 143, 145
and communication skills, 70
cross-cultural studies of, 61
delaying, 12
discussed in group sessions, 108–109, 110
high-risk, 49–53, 56
modification of, 54–56
and reaching/counseling partners, 25, 26
substance use during, 56–57
unprotected, 22, 51, 52, 55–56
Sexual partner issues, information about, 207–208, 210–211; *see also* Women, as partners of injected drug users
Sexually transmitted diseases, education about, 174
Sharing, in drug culture, 29–31; *see also* Needle sharing
Shooting galleries, 9, 13, 31, 32, 66
and needle sharing, 72, 73, 169
Skills-building groups, 101, 103–104, 115
Social influences, in AIDS risk reduction, 65

Social support, 70–71, 94, 118
Sociocultural variables, 63, 72–73
Spermicides, 12, 106, 124
Stigmatized groups, 23, 24–25, 26–27, 56, 59–60, 168
Stimulants, injectable, 7
  treatment for abuse of, 86–87
"Stop AIDS" movement, 114
Stress, AIDS-related, 92
Suicidal behavior, 84, 90, 93–94
"Survival" kits, 105, 109, 114, 125
Susceptibility, perceived, 64, 65, 66, 68, 117, 125
  and anxiety, 71, 118
Syphilis, 32
Syringes
  access to, 122
  cleaning of, 106, 123
  exchange of, 13, 176
  single-use, 11
  as source of infection, 10

T

Therapeutic communities, 80–81, 103; *see also* Residential treatment program
Thrush infection, 25
Transmission, of HIV, 4, 6
  heterosexual, 6, 9, 15–16, 23, 44, 45, 48–49, 130
  limited to stigmatized groups, 23
  male-to-female vs. female-to-male, 48
"Twelve Step" programs, 79–80, 84, 173

U

Urine testing, 26, 82, 87, 95

V

Valdiserri, R. O. (quoted), 20
Visual aids, 108, 110, 117, 118, 124

W

Walden House (San Francisco), 80
Withdrawal, drug, 69, 122
Women
  beliefs about AIDS in, 132, 128
  and condom use, 52–53, 57–58, 109, 117, 124, 133–134, 140–142, 178
  counseling for, 130–149
  deaths of, 23, 131
  HIV infection in, 6, 9, 15–16, 23, 44, 46, 48, 130
  increase in AIDS in, 23, 130
  minority, 31, 45, 53, 59, 96, 130–131
  outpatient programs for, 101, 136, 174
  as partners of injected drug users, 52, 54, 56, 59, 130–149, 178
  poverty in, 9, 130, 132, 149
  in prostitution, 23, 50, 53, 131
  role of in drug culture, 30
  and sexual activity, 12, 23, 48, 50, 73, 178
  support services for, 140

Y

Youth Environment Services (San Francisco), 38

Z

Zidovudine (AZT), 4, 83

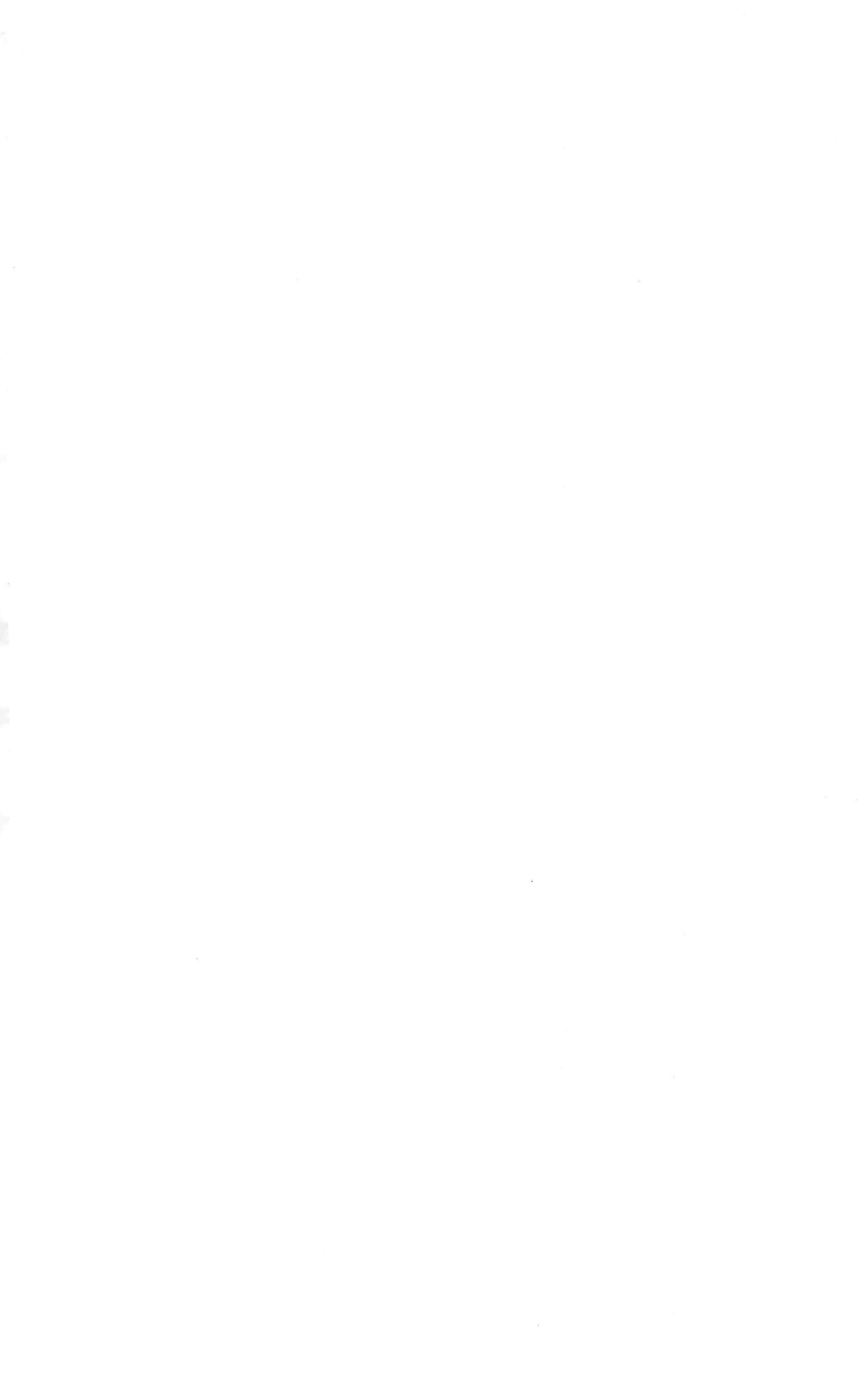